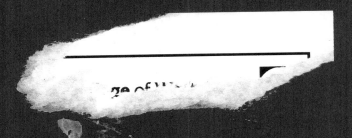

...ge of Wi...

...ANGLIA

...NTRE

NATIONAL CHILDBIRTH TRUST

COMPLETE BOOK OF
BABY CARE

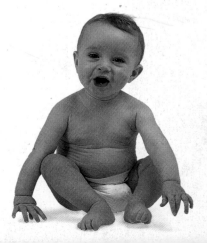

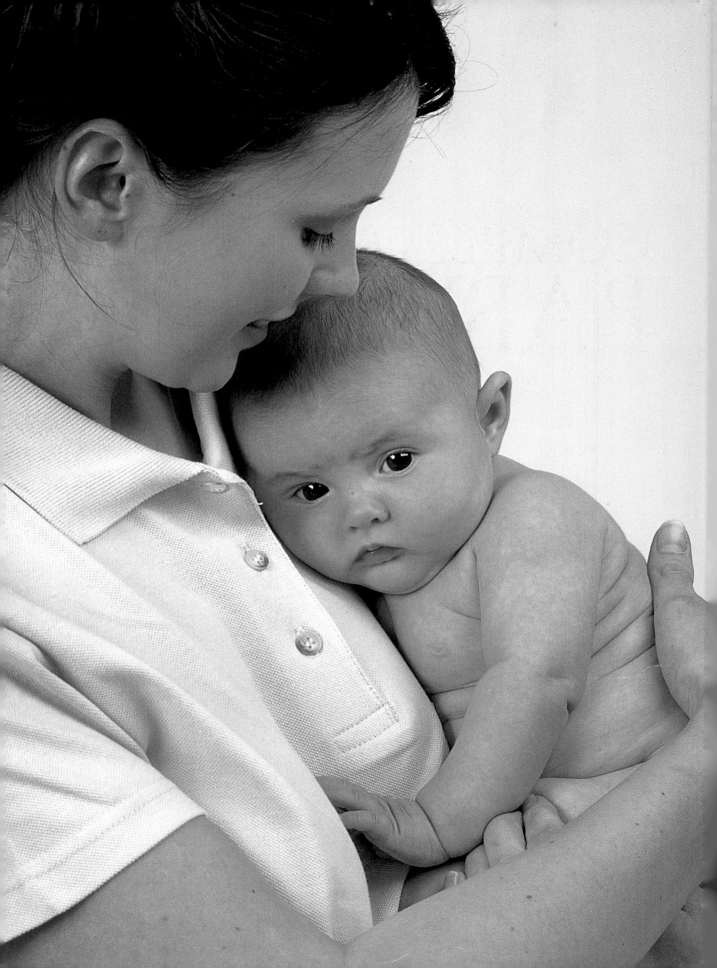

NATIONAL CHILDBIRTH TRUST

COMPLETE BOOK OF
BABY CARE

Edited by Daphne Metland
Photography by Anne Green-Armytage
Foreword by Fiona Phillips

Published by HarperCollins*Publishers* Ltd
in collaboration with
National Childbirth Trust Publishing

*The National Childbirth Trust (NCT) offers
information and support in pregnancy, childbirth
and early parenthood. We aim to give every
parent the chance to make informed choices. We
try to make sure that our services, activities and
membership are fully accessible to everyone.
Donations to support our work are welcome.*

*National Childbirth Trust, Alexandra House,
Oldham Terrace, London W3 6NH
Tel: 0181 992 8637*

ACKNOWLEDGEMENTS

Thank you to Gymboree (UK) Ltd for supplying us with
babywear and children's clothes and also Land's End and
Blooming Marvellous for loaning the adult outfits.
Equipment pictured is all available from IKEA and toys
from the Early Learning Centre. Wilkinet supplied the
baby sling, and all towels are by Christy. Disposable
nappies by Pampers; reusables by Zorbit and Mikey Diaper.

Thank you, too, to all the real parents and children who
kindly obliged when we asked them to come along and be
photographed just being gorgeous!

PICTURE ACKNOWLEDGEMENTS

Original photography by Anne Green-Armytage
© NCT Publishing
Additional photography:
George Williams pages 91, 127, 129, 137, 154, 159,
160, 180, 185, 201, 215 © NCT Publishing
Tony Sheffield/Phyll Buchanan page 25
Michael Bassett pages 62, 117
John Cocking/Telegraph Colour Library page 12
Anthea Sieveking/Collections page 12

Published by HarperCollins*Illustrated,* an imprint of
HarperCollins*Publishers* Ltd,
77–85 Fulham Palace Road, Hammersmith,
London W6 8JB
in collaboration with National Childbirth Trust
Publishing, 25–27 High Street, Chesterton,
Cambridge CB4 IND, UK

© 1999 NCT Publishing

A CIP catalogue record for this book is available from
the British Library.

ISBN 000 414053 2

Design by Tim McPhee
Editorial by Sonia Leach and Richard Westwood
Project Co-ordination by Debbie Wayment and
Jo'e Coleby

Production in association with Book Production
Consultants plc, 25–27 High Street, Chesterton,
Cambridge CB4 IND, UK

Printed and bound in Italy

THE AUTHORS

DAPHNE METLAND has prepared hundreds of couples for the birth of their babies through her 15 years' work as an antenatal teacher with the National Childbirth Trust. A consumer journalist by profession, she is a regular contributor to magazines, TV and radio. After taking a break to have two children, Daphne returned to full-time journalism as editor of *Parents* magazine and is now managing editor of NCT Publishing.

PENNEY HAMES, MA, trained first as a journalist and later as a clinical child psychologist. She deferred any practical application of either skill until after a lengthy research and development phase conducted on her own two children. Penney Hames has represented the NCT on the All Party Parliamentary Group on Parenting, and now combines writing with child guidance work.

MORAG MARTINDALE is a GP and family planning doctor working in Tayside. She has three children and joined the NCT during her second pregnancy. She is currently involved at a regional level as area representative for Tayside and Fife. She is also a member of the Tayside Joint Breastfeeding Initiative.

TERESA WILSON writes about parenting and health issues for a number of parenting journals. She also teaches on a Nursery Nurses training course at her local college in Berkshire. Her involvement with the NCT spans nine years, during which time she has been a breastfeeding counsellor and a postnatal discussion leader. She is now a national tutor in Postnatal Discussion. She has three children.

SUE ALLEN-MILLS is variously a mother, a writer and editor, and an NCT antenatal teacher, depending on what time of day it is. Before children, she was an editor of social science books. Since becoming a mother, she has worked as a writer and has been an NCT teacher since 1991.

Sue is married and lives in Cambridge with her two daughters, from whom she continues to learn about being a parent.

ANNE GREEN-ARMYTAGE worked as a computer consultant in the City of London before rediscovering her childhood love of photography after the birth of her first daughter. She now works as a freelance photographer part-time, concentrating on babies, plants and gardens, not necessarily in that order, for various magazines and books.

An active member of the NCT, Anne has been a newsletter editor, antenatal bookings clerk and chair of her local branch. She now has two daughters who occasionally agree, with much bribery and cajoling, to be photographed by their mother!

Publisher's note

All comments and personal accounts were given to us in confidence, so out of respect to our contributors' privacy we have changed all the names. We have endeavoured where possible to reproduce quotations verbatim, but where editing has been applied, the integrity of the quotation has been maintained.

The ages we have quoted in this book are a very rough guide to a baby's development. All babies are individual and of course your baby is special and will do things in his or her own way and in his or her own time. In the interests of equality, we have chosen to refer to the baby sometimes as 'he' and sometimes as 'she' in the text.

Editor's introduction

This book has grown out of the questions and comments of the many couples who have attended my National Childbirth Trust antenatal classes over the last decade and a half. All those new mums and dads told me very clearly what they wanted to find out from a babycare book: the real experiences of real parents. They didn't need another 'expert' handing down advice from on high, thank you very much. Instead, they wanted straight baby care information, the facts about child development, and how other new parents manage; everything they needed to know, in fact, to make up their own minds.

Many of those selfsame couples who attended my antenatal classes, also kindly agreed to be photographed here. My thanks go to all of these wonderful parents, and indeed all the people who have attended classes and in so doing have taught me so much about life as a new parent.

Daphne Metland
Editor

FOREWORD

By television presenter Fiona Phillips

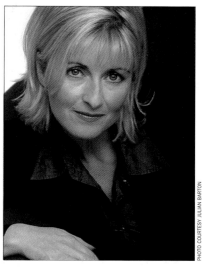

PHOTO COURTESY JULIAN BARTON

As I write this, I'm expecting my first baby. I'm aware that none of my clothes fit, I can't face coffee and I could happily sleep right round the clock if they let me! And I've only got another two months in which to learn all the basics of how to look after a baby.

Today's expectant mother has to schedule the birth in to a packed timetable that often includes career pressures, home-making demands and all sorts of wider family obligations coming at her from all directions. There have probably never been more demands made on our time and energy in the history of womankind ever before!

This means that we just don't have time for finding out the long way how to look after a baby: we want instant answers and quick results, which is where a book like this can come in handy. I need to know the quickest, most efficient way to change a nappy, put on a sling or soothe a crying baby.

I really like this book's easy-to-follow format, especially the checklists and chunks of summarised information. And I'm fascinated by the 'diary' sections, outlining a day in the life of a real baby at each of the stages covered. I like to look at these and think about what my baby will be like this time next year.

The National Childbirth Trust has been in existence, supporting parents for the last 40 years, and this book brings together the combined expertise and hands-on skills of all those mothers and fathers. But it's not going to tell you what to do; it tells you what other parents have done. It gives you the options, then leaves you to make up your own mind.

If, like me, you're facing first-time motherhood, this guide to the next three years will help enormously!

Fiona Phillips
X

CONTENTS

YOUR BABY FROM 0–1 MONTH

Newborn babies can do a lot: they can cry, look, listen, lift and turn their heads, grasp and wriggle, and, of course, they can suck. From birth, they're programmed to communicate.

Your newborn baby has many skills but some are simply reflexes. You shine a light in her eyes and she blinks, you stroke her cheek and she turns towards your finger. She's not clever, she just can't help herself. But she's amazing nonetheless. Without these involuntary responses to stimulation, she wouldn't survive. Some of these reflexes, like breathing and blinking, are permanent. Others, like stepping and the startle reflex give way to activities which are learnt, and others still, like tracking and sucking develop, through practise, into something more sophisticated and adaptable – something truly clever.

Babies want to understand, and feel happier when they do. But they don't have the ability to sit back and think. Babies learn by doing. Newborn babies actively look and listen. At the moment of birth a baby can follow a moving light with her eyes. A mere few hours later she begins to imitate facial expressions. During your first cuddle, try poking your tongue out at your baby, or raising your eyebrows up and down slowly and deliberately – she's likely to copy you unless she's very sleepy. For her, seeing something and doing it is one and the same thing. From the first, babies try to make sense of what's going on and act on the sense they make.

EARLY LEARNING

The way that you care for your baby allows her to gain the experience which will help her to develop. Being fed allows her to practise sucking. Having cuddles allows her to practise scanning your face with her eyes. And having a toy bobbed in front of her by her fascinated sister allows her to practise tracking and develop her idea of object constancy – the idea that things remain the same size no matter how near or far away they are.

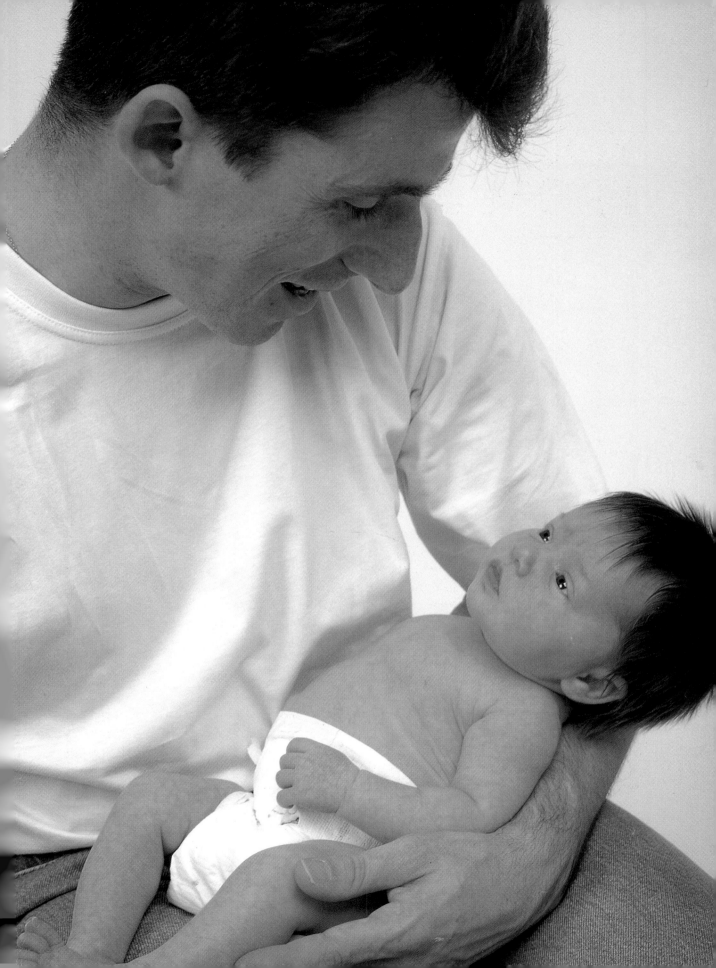

SOME OF YOUR NEWBORN BABY'S REFLEXES

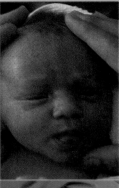

BLINK

Blinks when you clap your hands near her face

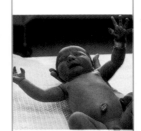

STARTLE OR 'MORO'

Throws out her legs and arms and arches her back if her head suddenly drops backwards

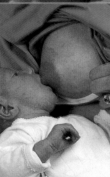

ROOTING

Turns her head towards your finger, or nipple, stroked against her cheek

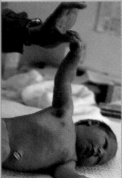

PALMAR

Closes her fist around anything which touches her palm

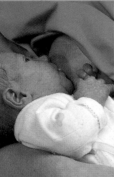

SUCKING

Sucks your finger or nipple rhythmically

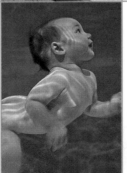

DIVING

Closes the tract to the lungs, keeps her mouth and eyes open and makes swimming movements with arms and legs when submerged under water

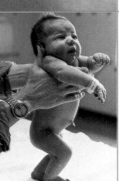

STEPPING

Makes walking movements when held upright with her feet touching a flat surface

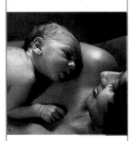

TRACKING

Follows moving objects with her eyes

Of course, these skills are not all that your baby learns. Skills develop within the context of a caring relationship. You care for your baby, and eventually your love will be reflected back. It is your baby's belief in herself, learnt from your belief in her, which motivates her desire to learn more. Love, praise and new experiences make learning new things secure, fun and exciting.

ATTACHMENT

Attachment is the name given to the relationship between a baby and her parents. In simple terms it is about love. Love doesn't come automatically with a baby. If it was that simple it wouldn't be such a big deal. Some parents fall head over heels as soon as their baby takes her first gasp, others wait for long, agonising months, only to be startled into it. Eye contact is important. Looking directly into each other's eyes can't help but make a connection. Skin-to-skin contact also triggers loving feelings.

Some experts used to feel that if you and your baby didn't have time together immediately after the birth then the chance to 'bond' would be lost. It's not so. For many reasons those first few minutes can be very precious, but if circumstances (caesarean birth, a baby who needs some medical help or whatever) make it impossible, don't panic. Nothing that cannot be gained later has been lost. Just spend time trying to get to know your baby.

Yet there may be a sensitive period for beginning the process of falling in love with your baby: a time within the first year when it's easier, or less complicated, to react spontaneously to her. Postnatal depression may prevent you from using this time. If you feel you may be depressed – tearful, anxious, guilty or irritable – do visit your GP. Your baby needs

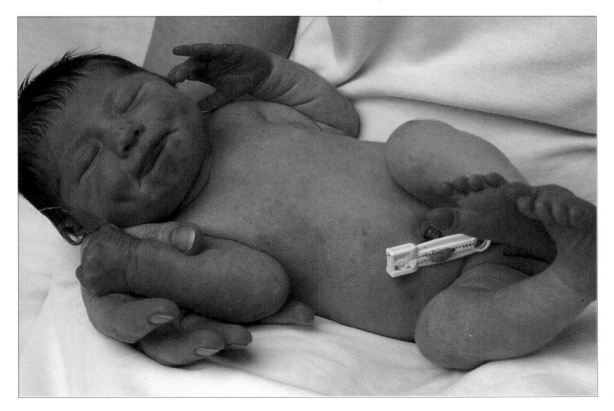

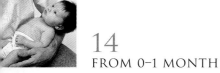
you to be there mentally as well as physically in order to begin this most important of relationships. She can't wait until your depression lifts, and nor should you.

RIGHT: Inside the womb, your baby was curled up snugly and it may take some time for her limbs to straighten. Her eyes can focus to a distance of about 20cm, and she will enjoy looking at your face

BELOW: Babies respond to sounds in the womb before birth and, once born, can tell the difference between their mother's voice and the voices of others

BOTTOM: It may take some time for your baby's circulation to establish itself. Hands and feet may look bluish at the beginning

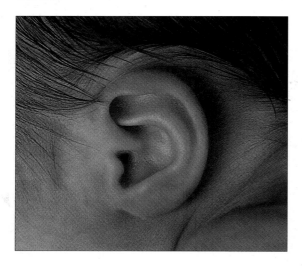

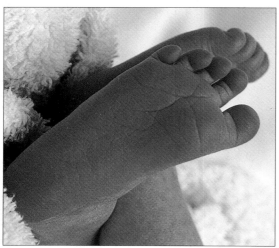

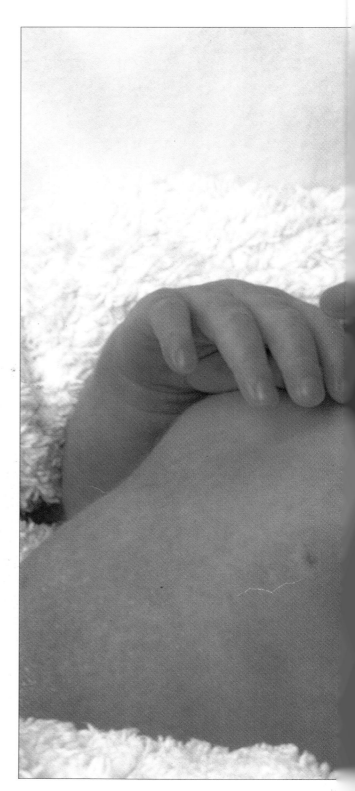

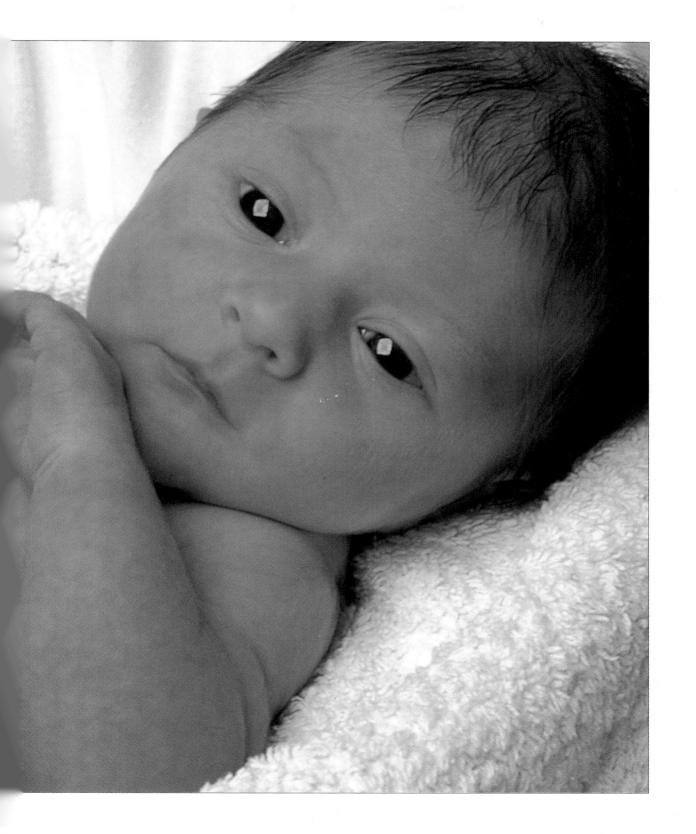

DIARY OF A NEWBORN

Isabella is 13 days old. Her father, Steve, works from home, and her mother, Sarah, is on maternity leave, so both of them are at home at the moment.

Sarah and Steve have found that 'everything has been thrown up in the air' since Isabella was born. 'Life as we knew it has gone out of the window,' says Steve. 'We don't seem to achieve much, but we're incredibly busy.'

7am

Isabella wakes up and has a long feed, lasting for about an hour.

8am

They all go back to sleep.

10–10.30am

Steve gets up, showers and gets dressed while Sarah feeds Isabella. Then Steve looks after Isabella while Sarah gets up. 'I love seeing her smile,' he says. 'I know they say babies don't smile at this age, but she *does*!' He also enjoys having long periods of eye contact with her.

11.30am

Breakfast for Sarah and Steve. Steve then takes the dog out, while Sarah potters at home.

1pm

Isabella has another feed. She wants to feed almost every hour during the afternoon and is usually awake between feeds. Sarah says, 'I spend hours and hours

breastfeeding. I feel like a milk-dispensing machine.' Steve is looking forward to the time when he can feed Isabella some expressed breast milk. 'Milk is Isabella's main need at the moment, and I can't give her that, so I feel rather as if I'm the less-important parent,' he says. Sarah doesn't agree, saying that Steve does other important things for Isabella, like changing her nappy, talking to her and cuddling her. He's also keeping the household running – doing the cooking, washing up, washing, and looking after the dog.

5pm

Isabella sleeps for a couple of hours. Sarah and Steve use this time to be together and 'try and be a bit normal'. They talk over things they're concerned about, or read or watch television. Sometimes, though, they use the time to have a nap. They're averaging about five hours' sleep a night, and they're both unbelievably tired. Steve speaks of experiencing 'a level of

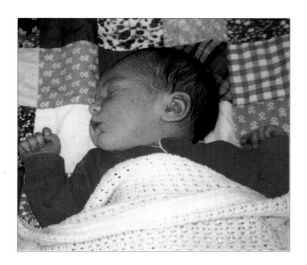

exhaustion second to none in my whole life'. They worry about how they'll cope with this lack of sleep and how long it will go on for. 'I dream of having four hours' uninterrupted sleep,' says Sarah.

7pm
Isabella wakes and has another feed, then goes back to sleep. She hasn't had a bath today. Sarah and Steve have given her two baths since she was born but they haven't gone very well. 'I think maybe we didn't time it right,' says Sarah. But despite the lack of success with baths, Sarah and Steve are becoming more skilled at the practical aspects of babycare. 'We've learnt that the important thing is to be very prepared, and to have everything you need to hand. It's also important not to panic if something goes wrong, because then Isabella panics. The more relaxed you are, the better it is for the baby.'

8pm
Isabella sleeps while Sarah and Steve have supper. She wakes for another feed during the evening.

11pm
Sarah and Steve go to bed.

12.30am
Isabella wakes for a feed.

3am
Isabella wakes again for a feed.

One major change that Sarah and Steve have found since Isabella was born is that they can't make plans any more. Everything has to fit around Isabella. 'She's in charge,' says Steve. Nor is it possible for them to be spontaneous. 'We can't just say "let's go out for dinner" or go to the cinema, or even have a long shower!' says Sarah. They're glad that they bought what they needed for Isabella and stocked up on food and household essentials before Isabella was born, because there's no time for that now. Sarah says she wonders if she'll ever go out again. But they don't mind these constraints because Isabella is so rewarding.

There are moments of anxiety too, however. They worry about whether Isabella is being fed too much or too little, if she's too hot or too cold, if her nappy is being changed often enough, if she's getting enough or too much stimulation, if she's breathing. 'It's instant anxiety on all fronts,' says Sarah. 'The responsibility is overwhelming.'

Sarah says that being a parent is twice as good as she expected and twice as difficult. 'I had an idea what it would be like because I have younger siblings who were born when I was a teenager, but it's one thing to know it in theory and another to actually go through it.' Steve says that he had no expectations, which increases the wonder of parenthood, as well as the shock of it.

They feel that they're coping well, and say that they're lucky to have an excellent support network, to have both of them at home, and that their daughter Isabella is such a lovely sweet-tempered baby.

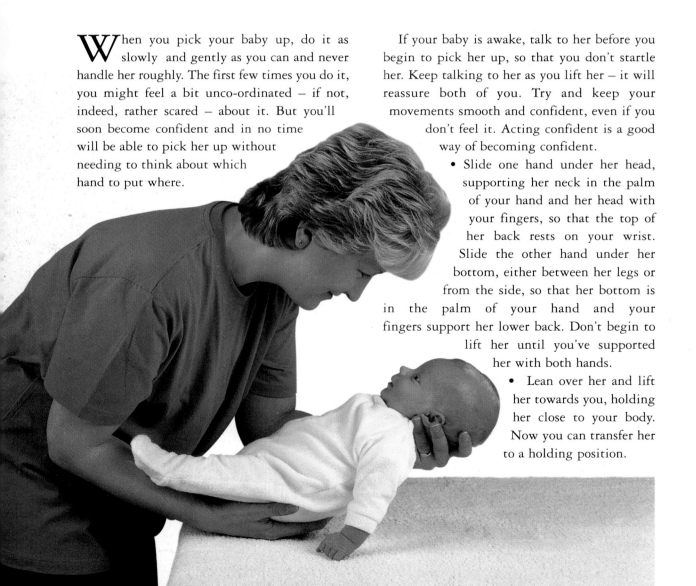
HOLDING YOUR BABY

New babies can seem as if they're very fragile and will easily break. They're not and they won't. Holding your baby firmly and securely (as she was held in the womb) won't hurt her. On the contrary, it'll reassure her. She particularly needs to have her head firmly supported until her neck muscles develop and she's able to do this for herself. Although it won't seriously harm her if her head is allowed to flop, she'll think she's going to be dropped and that will alarm her.

When you pick your baby up, do it as slowly and gently as you can and never handle her roughly. The first few times you do it, you might feel a bit unco-ordinated – if not, indeed, rather scared – about it. But you'll soon become confident and in no time will be able to pick her up without needing to think about which hand to put where.

If your baby is awake, talk to her before you begin to pick her up, so that you don't startle her. Keep talking to her as you lift her – it will reassure both of you. Try and keep your movements smooth and confident, even if you don't feel it. Acting confident is a good way of becoming confident.

• Slide one hand under her head, supporting her neck in the palm of your hand and her head with your fingers, so that the top of her back rests on your wrist. Slide the other hand under her bottom, either between her legs or from the side, so that her bottom is in the palm of your hand and your fingers support her lower back. Don't begin to lift her until you've supported her with both hands.

• Lean over her and lift her towards you, holding her close to your body. Now you can transfer her to a holding position.

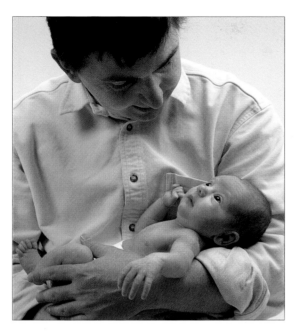

HOLDING YOUR BABY

• On your shoulder

Many parents find that this is a good position for soothing a crying or fretful baby, or for carrying a sleepy baby.

Lift your baby to your shoulder, so that her body is upright and her head is resting on your shoulder. You can either leave the hand that was supporting her head in the same place or bring it across so that it encircles her upper back. With your other hand, support her bottom. Hold her firmly, so that she feels secure.

There are all kinds of variations on this hold. Once you've put your baby to your shoulder you can switch hands – easier than it sounds – so that the hand that was supporting her head supports her bottom and vice versa. As you become more confident, you'll find that you can hold your baby in this position one-handed too.

New mum, Sarah, comments: 'I love the feeling of Adam nuzzling into my neck. He makes these lovely little snuffly noises.'

• Cradling

Cradling your baby is a good position for rocking her, and excellent for looking at her and talking or singing to her.

Hold your baby in your arms, so that her head rests just above the crook of your arm, with your lower arm supporting her body and her upper leg resting in your hand. Your other hand goes under her bottom. Hold her so that she's lying with her head slightly higher than her bottom.

With practice, you'll find that you can hold your baby in this position using just one arm, supporting her bottom with that hand. This leaves your other hand free to do such essential other things as eating your lunch.

'I could spend hours just holding Eleanor in my arms and looking at her face,' says one dad.

HOLDING YOUR OLDER BABY

When your baby is older and has more control over her head and neck, you can hold her facing forwards with her back against your chest, or with her sitting astride your hip. Both these positions are excellent for letting her see what's going on in the world.

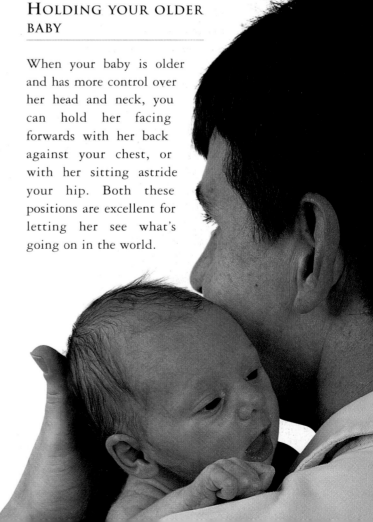

STEP BY STEP SWADDLING

Swaddling is an age-old method of soothing an unsettled or distressed baby. Some babies simply won't go to sleep unless they're securely wrapped up. For others, it can be a way of giving them the feeling of being held while giving you the chance to do something with your arms free – like get dressed, for example!

Not all babies like to be swaddled, but if yours does, it can be a good way of calming her. Some babies like to be swaddled with both their arms wrapped up. Others – especially those who've discovered that they like sucking their fist – will want to have a hand left free to suck. You'll soon discover what your baby prefers.

If you're swaddling your baby to comfort her when she's crying, you may have to cope with flailing arms and legs. Hold her arms gently with one hand as you wrap the sheet round her with the other. This will require you to swap hands as you bring the second side of the sheet (step 3) over the baby (it's not as tricky as it sounds).

Be careful not to overwrap your baby, or she could become overheated, especially in a warm house. If you swaddle her to sleep, it's better to use a cot sheet rather than a blanket, and don't put

many more blankets on top of her – maybe one, if that, in the summer and two or three in the winter, depending on the temperature of your house. (See box on right.)

1 Spread a cot sheet or cotton blanket on a flat surface. You can leave it open, or fold it in half to form a triangle, whichever you prefer. You won't be able to form a perfect triangle if your sheet is rectangular, but your baby won't mind. Lay your baby on the top of the sheet with the back of her neck in line with the long edge.

For the first month or two, she'll probably lie with her arms bent at the elbow so that her hands are up by her shoulders and with her knees bent up towards her body. That's fine – there's no need to try and straighten her out.

2 Bring one side of the sheet diagonally across her shoulder and tuck it under her body, leaving her arm on that side free. You may need to roll her slightly onto her side in order to do this. The sheet should be snug around her, but not too tight.

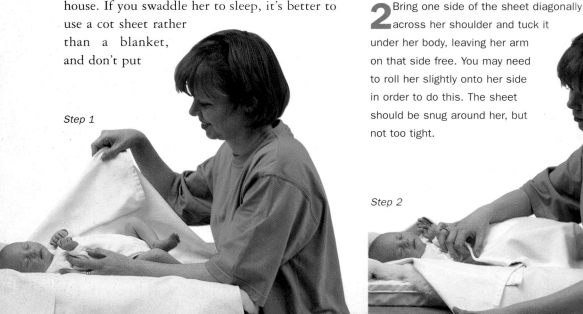

Step 1

Step 2

3 Then bring the remaining side across her uncovered shoulder and tuck that under the other side of her body.

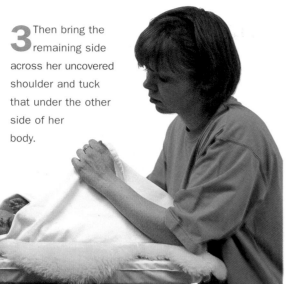

4 You can tuck the bottom end of the sheet up under her feet to make it warm and cosy if you want to, or you can leave it loose, if you prefer. Your baby will now feel nice and secure.

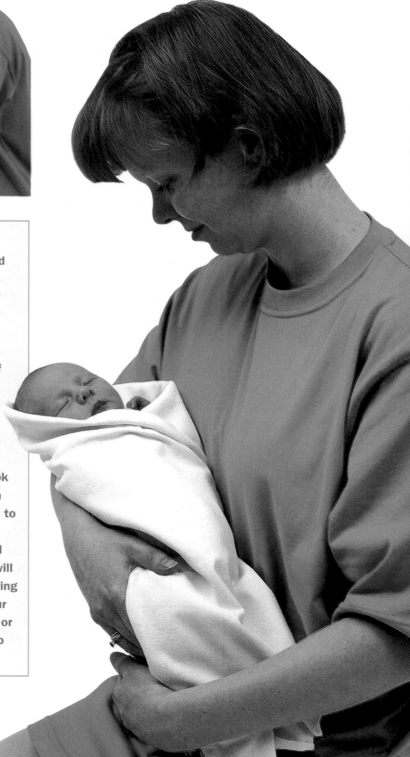

TOO HOT OR TOO COLD?

Your baby's hands and feet aren't a good guide to her temperature. They may feel cold to the touch – and in the very early days may even look blue – even though she's quite warm enough.

The best way to check whether she's too hot or too cold is to feel the back of her neck or her chest, underneath her clothing. Her skin should feel as warm as, or slightly warmer than, your hand.

A baby who's too hot will feel sweaty or clammy and may have a heat rash, especially around her neck. She may look red in the face and may cry. Removing a layer of clothing or bedding will help her to cool down.

A baby who's too cold may shiver and cry. A baby who has become very cold will be very still, however, because she's trying to conserve energy to keep warm. If your baby is too cold, add a layer of clothing or bedding, or hold her next to your body to warm her up.

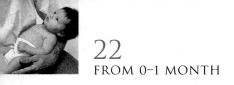

CHOOSING HOW TO FEED YOUR BABY

Looking at the summary opposite, it is clear to see that breastfeeding has many advantages for babies, and these last well into later life, too, with less respiratory illness, for example, among children who were breastfed as babies. Many mothers also derive a great deal of pleasure from breastfeeding, both physical and emotional, although some do find it tiring to start with or difficult to get into practice. If you decide to feed your baby yourself, talk to your midwife, health visitor, or your local NCT breastfeeding counsellor. And get a good book on breastfeeding before your baby is born, so you know what to expect.

BREAST AND FORMULA MILKS

Formula milk is based on cow's milk protein, rather than human protein. Changes are being made all the time, but it is unlikely there will ever be any real comparison in terms of quality of milk for human babies. Because breast milk

FEEDING EQUIPMENT

FOR BREASTFEEDING:
(Only breasts and baby are really essential for breastfeeding, but these items will help make it more comfortable and convenient.)

● FEEDING BRAS
You'll need at least two. Make sure that they open fully, are properly fitted and don't press into you anywhere. A wide adjustment round the chest is useful.

● BREAST PADS
Slip inside your bra and act as blotting paper for leaking milk.

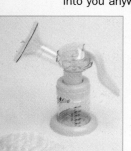

● BREAST PUMPS
If your breasts are engorged, or you'd like someone else to feed your baby, you may need to express milk. You can do this by hand, but it can be easier with a breast pump. A large variety is now available: electric, battery and hand operated. Whichever one you choose, give it time while you learn to use it effectively. As it must be sterilised, look for one that is easy to reassemble.

● BREAST SHELLS
Hard plastic shells that you put inside your bra to collect milk from the other breast when you are feeding or expressing. They should only be used when you are feeding, and need sterilising regularly.

● BREAST CREAMS
Creams aim to reduce nipple soreness and usually contain soothing agents such as calendula. They may offer some relief, but if your nipples are sore, this may be due to poor positioning and you may prefer to seek advice from a midwife or breastfeeding counsellor.

● NIPPLE SHIELDS
A soft rubber nipple-cover that can relieve soreness in the short term – as long as the baby then accepts the naked nipple later on and is not shield dependent.

changes its composition as the baby grows, and because of the immunological and antibacterial benefits that it confers, it simply cannot be copied by formula manufacturers.

KEEPING AN OPEN MIND

Many new mothers change their minds about feeding their baby after the birth. Often, breastfeeding is much easier than anticipated, and it can also give closeness with their baby that is very enjoyable. Some mothers find that they just don't like it, and opt for bottle-feeding. It is important to feel comfortable with the decision that you have made.

It's very difficult to reverse a decision to bottle-feed from the beginning, so many experts recommend giving breastfeeding a try for the first few days if you're undecided.

FOR BOTTLE-FEEDING:

- BOTTLES

You'll need at least six bottles with teats and caps.

- STERILISING EQUIPMENT

All bottle-feeding equipment must be sterilised after use. This can range from the microwave sterilising system, easy to use, to a large, emptied ice cream tub with sterilising tablets added to the water.

- LONG-HANDLED BRUSH

Bottle-feeding equipment needs to be cleaned thoroughly before sterilising.

- INFANT MILK

There are a number of brands available. Check your choice with your midwife or health visitor. For convenience, some infant milk is sold already made up – an expensive option but very useful for days out.

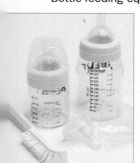

BREASTFEEDING OR BOTTLE-FEEDING?

BREASTFEEDING

- The quality of the milk is nutritionally superior and changes as the baby grows to meet all her needs.
- There is less chance of developing allergies.
- Breast milk contains antibodies which give distinct health benefits.
- Breast milk is free, needing only a small amount of extra food for you.
- There is no preparation time, and no need for sterilisation.
- Breast milk is specifically made for human babies – it is the best possible food for them, helping development of the brain and nervous systems, and protecting against gastrointestinal and middle ear problems.
- Research indicates that breastfeeding is also beneficial for mothers, giving some protection against certain forms of cancer and osteoporosis.
- Breast milk is always delivered at exactly the right temperature.

BOTTLE-FEEDING

- The responsibility for feeding can be shared between the parents and other carers more equally.
- Some people think that bottle-fed babies sleep for longer than their breastfed counterparts, and there is evidence to support this.
- The amount that the baby takes in a feed can be measured.
- There is no change of feeding method if you are returning to work.

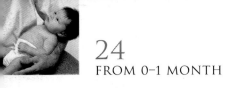

HOW BREASTFEEDING WORKS

All through pregnancy, your breasts will have been preparing for lactation and you will start making milk for your baby as soon as you have given birth and the placenta is delivered.

As your baby suckles, your body's hormonal response (called the 'let down reflex') is to draw the milk down inside your breast so that it collects behind the areola. Hormones alert the body when more milk needs to be made, as well as squeezing the milk out of the milk-producing

'My partner came to antenatal classes with me, so he knew how breastfeeding worked as well. I found it very useful because he reminded me of the bits I'd forgotten.'

cells in your breasts, in response to your baby suckling. Sometimes you will see milk squirting from one or more of the many pin-sized openings in the nipple as the let down happens.

You may also feel a tingling sensation in your breasts and sometimes a sense of calmness and

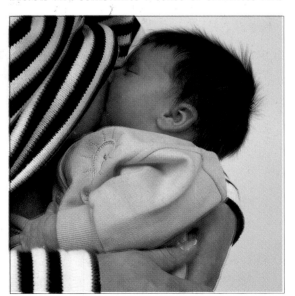

relaxation as you settle back to enjoy the feed.

Sometimes, at the beginning of a feed, you may feel your uterus contract, which can feel like a mild contraction or a period pain. This is also the work of hormones, and the pain will stop very soon after the birth. It is doing you good because it means that your uterus is returning to its original size. Take a paracetamol 20 minutes or so before a feed, if the pain is very uncomfortable.

BABY-LED FEEDING

After one or two days, when your baby takes a feed, your body responds by making more milk to replace what has gone. This supply and demand system means that the more your baby feeds, the more milk you will make.

Whatever your baby's appetite, you will be able to make enough milk. If she seems to be hungry all the time she may be having a growth spurt, or you may need to check with your health visitor or breastfeeding counsellor that she is properly latched on. If she is not well latched on, your nipples could be getting sore.

Let your baby set the pace for feeding. By letting her feed on demand, your body will respond by producing the correct supply for her. If you try to restrict the length of feeds, you won't make the right amount of milk. Similarly, if you top up with formula milk because you don't think you are making enough yourself,

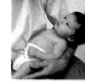

JAUNDICE

Some infants develop jaundice after birth and will look yellow (even suntanned) and be sleepy. This is usually because the baby's immature liver can't work efficiently at first.

If this happens, try giving your baby frequent breastfeeds – around 12 a day – waking the baby if necessary. The breast milk will help your baby pass more motions, speeding up the elimination of the waste product, bilirubin.

You may also be offered phototherapy, a light treatment that speeds up recovery. Ask your midwife for more information.

---

your own supply will diminish accordingly.

It may seem that you're feeding a lot in the first weeks, but you will reap the rewards very quickly. As the baby grows, she will become more efficient and therefore quicker, at feeding. Her stomach will be growing all the time too, enabling her to take in more milk at each feed. The main thing is that the two of you will get better at it as you work together.

CHANGING MILK: THE FIRST DAYS

You can offer a feed as soon as you and your baby are ready. It can be a good idea to feed in the first hour after birth – it gives closeness and will fill your baby to keep hunger at bay for the next few hours. Don't worry if she doesn't want to feed straight away; she will when the time is right. She may be quite tired for the first 24 to 48 hours, particularly if you were given pethidine during your labour.

Colostrum, the first fluid your breasts produce, provides protection for your baby until her own immune system can start functioning.

Colostrum is low in volume but very high in protein, antibodies, vitamins and anti-infective agents. Your baby will be getting this perfectly balanced nourishment for the first two or three days, until your mature breast milk 'comes in'. Don't worry if she doesn't appear to feed very much for the first day or so. Her stomach is still very small, and the nutrients in colostrum are very much concentrated.

(If your baby arrives early, your body will produce a milk particularly rich in essential nutrients and proteins, just right for a premature baby. Over time, this will adjust until it's tailor-made for a two-, three-, or even a 30-month baby.)

Once the mature milk has arrived, with its perfect balance of proteins, carbohydrates, fats, vitamins and minerals, your baby will first get foremilk. This is a thirst-quenching drink high in lactose (sugar) but low in fat. As the feed progresses, hindmilk is released with the let down reflex. Hindmilk is higher in fat content and is important for the baby's growth.

For this reason, do clear one breast before offering the other one, so that she benefits from the high fat content at the end of the meal.

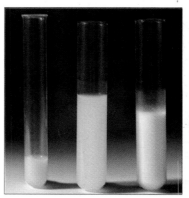

EXPRESSED BREAST MILK (left to right)
COLOSTRUM: An amazingly rich mixture of proteins, vitamins, and anti-infective agents designed to help a newborn through the first days of life
FOREMILK: Watery, but full of lactose sugar
HINDMILK: Loaded with fats and calories; the part of a feed which really satisfies a hungry baby

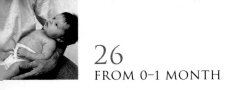

LATCHING ON GUIDE

Make sure that you feel comfortable before you start to feed your baby. Being physically relaxed will ease the whole process, so it's worth making a few preparations in advance.

When you are getting ready to feed your baby, make sure that she is lying on her side, facing you. She should be tucked in closely to your body, with her head resting on your forearm. Her nose should be opposite your nipple, and she should be the same height as the nipple, probably lying on pillows.

If you gently touch your baby's mouth with your nipple, she will respond immediately by turning towards the touch and opening her mouth. This is the 'rooting reflex'. When she does this, she's ready for you to start feeding her.

RIGHT FROM THE START

As your baby opens her mouth wide, move her towards you so that she takes as much of the

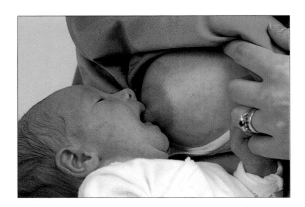

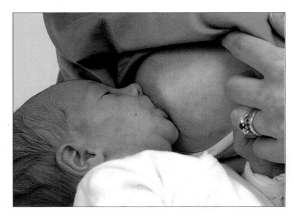

breast into her mouth as possible. Her tongue should be under your breast. If you feel a lot of pain, or your breast slips out of her mouth, take her off and start again. Keep trying until you get it right and you can feel that she is firmly on.

FINISHING A FEED

Insert your little finger inside your baby's mouth, between your breast and the corner of

CHECKLIST:

- choose a chair that supports you well, particularly your back and shoulders
- have pillows or cushions to support your back, and put one on your lap to bring your baby up to the same level as your breasts
- keep a drink close by: many mothers find breastfeeding makes them very thirsty
- make sure there's a snack close by
- take the phone off the hook, or put it on answerphone mode
- keep a book or the television remote to hand, so if the baby takes a long time, you won't have to move at all.

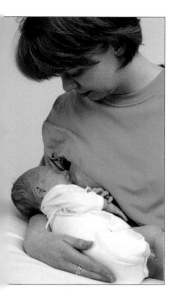

her mouth. This will break the suction and stop her from making you sore as she comes off.

It takes a little time for feeding patterns to develop. Offer your baby the breast whenever she wants it, and offer both breasts at every feed for now, although you should let her finish one side before offering her the other. If you don't do this, she may take in too much foremilk and not get enough of the nutritious hindmilk.

Don't time her feeds. She may fall asleep at the breast, so you can take her off gently and let her sleep – and don't worry too much if she doesn't want both breasts.

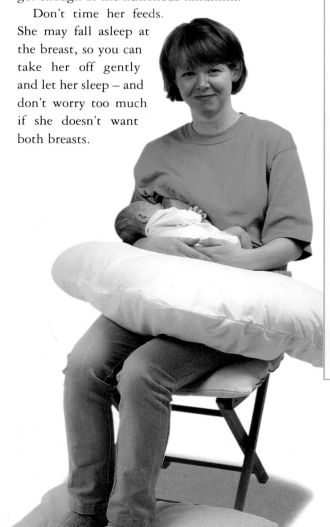

WHAT YOU SHOULD SEE
- baby tucked in close to you
- chin against breast, stretched upwards rather than tucked in
- wide open mouth, with bottom lip curled outwards
- face and jaw movement, maybe ear waggling
- lower lip taking more of areola than top lip

WHAT YOU SHOULDN'T SEE
- cheeks sucked in
- lips looking like sucking on a straw

WHAT YOU SHOULD HEAR
- some slow, some quick, sounds of milk being swallowed

WHAT YOU SHOULDN'T HEAR
- clicking noises
- lip smacking

WHAT YOU MAY FEEL
- a feeling of being 'firmly gripped'
- the let down reflex, a tingling sensation in the breasts, often at the beginning of a feed, as the milk starts to flow
- a fleeting pain at the start of a feed in the first few weeks

WHAT YOU SHOULDN'T FEEL
- pain which lasts throughout a feed

If you see, hear, or feel anything that you shouldn't, gently take the baby off and re-position her.

FEEDING POSITIONS

Whichever position you use, it is important to be comfortable, supported and relaxed throughout a breastfeed. This may mean a little preparation beforehand with pillows, cushions and finding a comfortable chair.

There is no end to the number of feeding positions you can adopt and the best ones are those that feel right to you. You may prefer to stick with one position until you become adept at breastfeeding. On the other hand, if you are finding things painful, a change of position sometimes makes all the difference. Even moving your baby a few centimetres up or down may help. Often mothers start to experiment as their confidence grows.

'For most of the time I used the classic position, but when I got sore I used the underarm one.'

helps to cup his head in your hand (left hand for right breast; right hand for left breast, obviously).

REMEMBER:

• Always make sure that your baby is facing the breast: that is, nose opposite nipple. It makes feeding more of an effort for him if he has to turn his head.
• Check that his ear, shoulder and hip are all in a line. He shouldn't be twisted round.
• Tuck him in closely to you.

Traditional position
He is supported by pillows on your lap, on the same level as your breasts, his head supported by your forearm, rather than in the crook of the arm, and his body lying across your stomach. Sometimes it

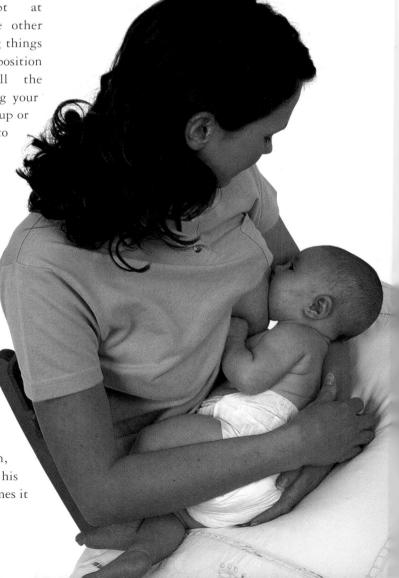

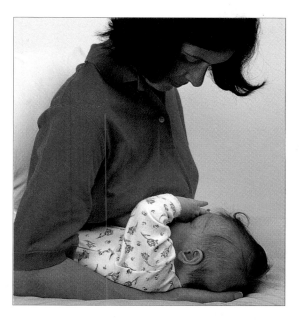

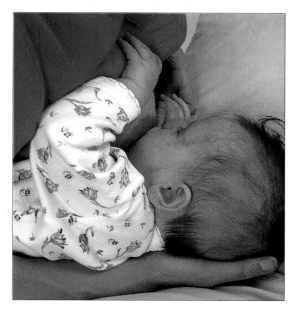

Underarm position

By placing cushions at your side, your baby can rest on them with his legs pointing behind you. Your arm enfolds him, and your right hand cradles his head as he feeds from your right breast (and vice versa). This position is sometimes used by women who have given birth by caesarean section, as it avoids pressure on a caesarean scar.

In the closer view above, you can see that the baby has a good mouthful of breast and is well latched on. He is able to suck without twisting his neck because head and body are lying in a straight line.

To make sure you're comfortable, always bring the baby to the breast with a good supporting cushion, not the breast to the baby.

Lying down

By lying on your side and resting your head on a pillow, your baby can tuck in close to you. He will have the support of the bed, and you can guide him to your breast and support him with your free hand. You may find that it helps to have a pillow behind your back to prevent backache. A thin pillow or large folded towel under your rib cage will lift your body slightly – helpful if you have large breasts.

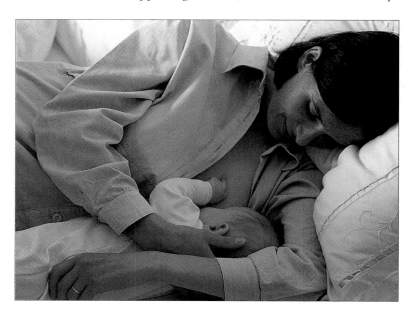

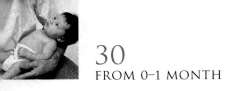

TROUBLESHOOTING: BREASTFEEDING PROBLEMS

SYMPTOMS:	Baby wants to feed all the time	Sore/cracked/bleeding nipples	Full, hard, lumpy breasts. Flattened nipples that make it difficult for the baby to latch on	Small lump in your breast, which is tender
CAUSES:	Poor positioning or a delay in your supply building up	Poor positioning Baby sucking on nipple rather than on breast	Primary engorgement, which often takes place when your milk first 'comes in' on the third or fourth day. Secondary engorgement, which happens when your baby drops a feed, perhaps when he first starts sleeping longer through the night. Your body will adjust to this quickly	Blocked duct: something has stopped the milk from flowing freely, and a blockage has been caused. This can happen if a bra is too tight, if you have sat for some hours with a seat belt across your breasts, or even if you have slept awkwardly
REMEDIES:	In the early weeks, your baby may simply be the kind who draws enormous comfort from the breast and wants to be there, sucking, all the time. If this is a change of pattern, though, your baby may be building up your milk supply. He should settle again in 24–48 hours. Let him feed on demand. If you are sore as well, your baby may not be positioned correctly. Ask your midwife to check that he is latched on properly	Take baby off (breaking grip with little finger first), and try again, making sure baby's mouth is wide open when she goes on. Ask someone to check the positioning for you. Also try different positions, such as holding her under your arm, or with you lying down to feed. TO RELIEVE SORENESS: Express a little milk and spread around nipples Feed from the least sore side first	Use warm flannels to help the milk to flow, or get into a bath or shower before feeding Express a little milk before offering your baby the breast, so that it is easier for him to latch on Feed your baby frequently to reduce fullness Put chilled Savoy cabbage leaves inside your bra (yes, seriously) to draw away the swelling	Use massage and warmth to help the milk to flow and disperse the lump Let your baby feed by positioning him with his lower jaw nearest to the lump, if possible so that the strong action of his jaw can 'feed it away' Feed from the sore side first Massage and express after a feed if your breast still feels full and lumpy

Breastfeeding is a skill that has to be learned by both mother and baby. For some, it can take a little while to settle down. Remember that every mother and baby pair is different and solutions that work for one, may not work for another.

Red, inflamed areas on breasts Flu-like symptoms: aching, temperature, weepy Full, sore breast	Sore nipples with white marks on them which don't heal/baby has white spots in mouth and nappy rash Deep breast pain after feeds	Baby won't take the breast
Mastitis: an inflammation of the breast, which happens when breast milk leaks into breast tissue	Thrush, which can sometimes occur after either you or your baby has a course of antibiotics, or may come out of the blue	Change of taste of breast milk, caused by change in diet, or course of tablets Using a nipple cream Stopping using nipple shields Periods starting/dental treatment/even hard exercise!
Go to bed and rest Continue to feed your baby, offering the sore side first Feed frequently Ask your midwife to recommend a painkiller Use warm and cold compresses to reduce swelling Contact your GP if you are worried, who will probably prescribe antibiotics	You should both be treated with an anti-fungal cream. Occasionally systemic medication is needed	Perseverance Try distraction – feeding standing up, in the bath, when your baby is half-asleep, or when the lights are dim If you want to stop using a nipple shield, trim it down with scissors, starting by snipping out the centre first. Cut off a little more each day. If breast refusal continues, you may need to express milk to keep up your milk supply.

HELP AVAILABLE

If you have a breastfeeding problem, aim to resolve it as quickly as possible. You can get help and support from:

- your midwife
- your health visitor
- an NCT breastfeeding counsellor
- the postnatal ward where you delivered your baby
- your GP
- your local NCT breast-feeding support group.

You don't have to join the National Childbirth Trust to get the help of one of their breastfeeding counsellors – anyone can contact them for support. You'll find the telephone number at the back of this book.

Do remember, though, that all the breastfeeding counsellors are volunteers with jobs and families of their own and that they may not always be able to visit you at home, but they can give suggestions over the phone. It can be reassuring to talk to someone experienced and fully trained, who has breastfed a baby herself, knows that setbacks can be overcome, and can well understand how you might be feeling.

STEP BY STEP
MAKING UP A BOTTLE

Today's formula milks have been developed so that they mimic the composition of breast milk as closely as possible. Be guided by your health visitor in your choice of powdered milk. She will help you choose the one most suitable for your newborn.

Make sure you read the instructions printed on the infant milk that you are about to use, carefully. The ratio of powder to water has been calculated in order to give your baby the right amount of nutrition.

'I enjoy giving Jack his bottle-feed in the early hours of the morning, while his mother is sleeping,' says Jim, Jack's dad

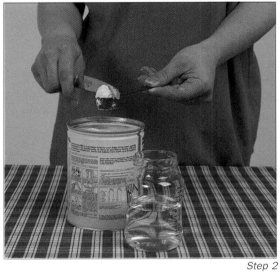
Step 2

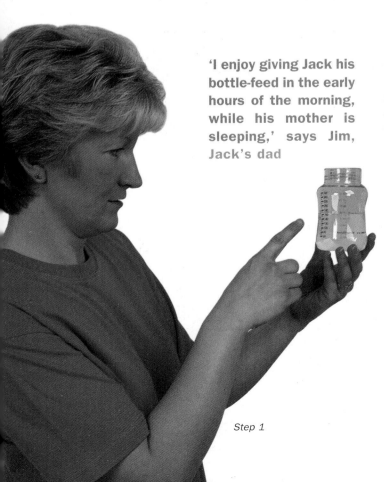
Step 1

1 Fill the bottle to the correct level of cooled boiled water. The simplest way to do this is to pour slightly more in, then tip some out until you have the right amount.

2 Using the scoop provided, take powder from the tin. Every time you take a scoop, level it off with a clean knife. Don't compress the powder.

3 Tip the powder into the bottle. This bit needs a steady hand, so don't wobble.

4 Put the top on the bottle and shake it thoroughly until all the powder is dissolved.

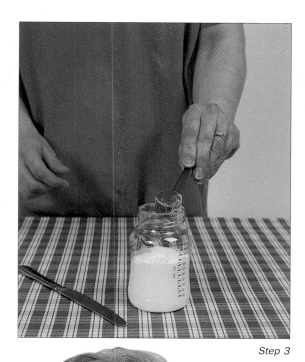

Step 3

STERILISING

All the equipment that you use to feed your baby must be washed and sterilised after use. Wash the bottles with a weak solution of detergent and a long-handled brush that can reach right to the bottom of the bottle. Make sure you rinse all the detergent out with clean water, then sterilise as below.

MICROWAVE STERILISING

- Pour the correct amount of water into the bottom of the steriliser.
- Place the tray containing bottles into the bottom section of the steriliser.
- Put the top on, place in the microwave and activate for the correct amount of time.

ALTERNATIVE STERILISING

You can also sterilise equipment in the following ways:
- boiling in water for at least ten minutes
- putting into a container with water and a sterilising tablet for a prescribed length of time
- using a steam steriliser.

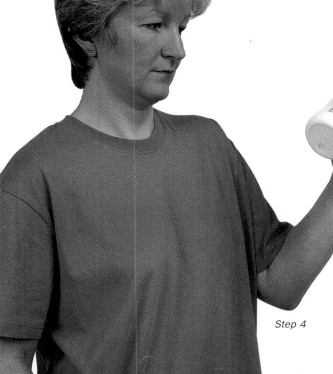

Step 4

MAKING UP A DAY'S FEEDS

- you can make up a bottle each time one is needed, or you can make up a whole day's feeds in one go
- made-up milk can be kept in the fridge for 24 hours
- when your baby needs feeding, take a bottle out of the fridge, and warm it by placing it in a jug of hot water.

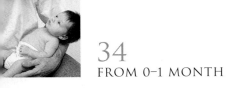
STEP BY STEP BOTTLE-FEEDING

*Your new baby will need several small feeds in a day at first –
about six to eight is typical. Because formula milk takes longer to
digest than breast milk, bottle-fed babies tend to feed less.*

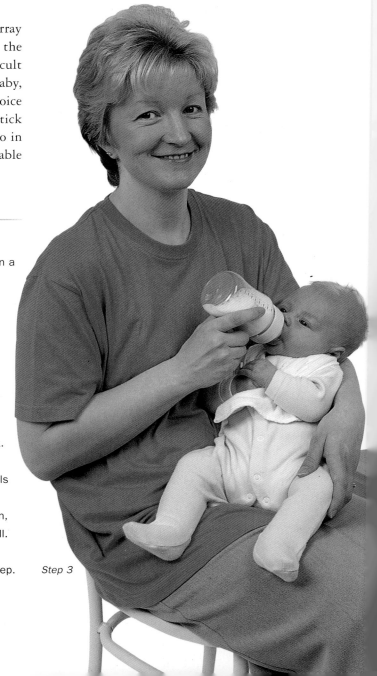

Step 3

You will be greeted by a bewildering array of formula milks when you visit the supermarket or chemist. It may seem difficult to know which one is best for your baby, especially if you are trying to make your choice before the birth. Many parents simply stick with the product that they are introduced to in hospital, but your health visitor should be able to help you make an informed choice.

GIVING THE BOTTLE

1 If you have taken the baby's bottle from the fridge, you should warm it for a few minutes in a jug of hot water. Make sure the milk isn't too hot by testing some on the back of your wrist.

2 Make sure you are sitting comfortably before you start feeding your baby.

3 Hold your baby in a semi-upright position on your lap, keeping her secure with your arm. With bottle-feeding, your baby doesn't need to be turned round towards you, but can lie on her back.

4 Keep the bottle tilted upwards so that milk fills the teat and no air bubbles can get into it. Otherwise your baby may get windy. Every so often, ease the teat out of her mouth, so that it can refill.

Once feeding time is over, your baby may fall asleep.

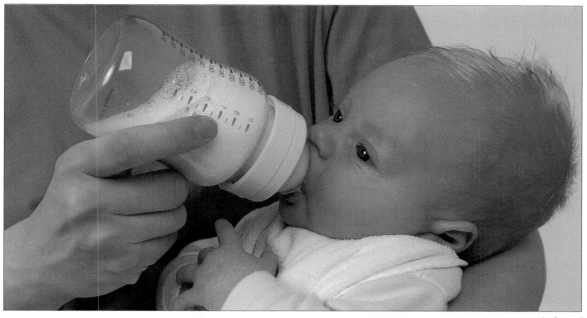

Step 4

WINDING METHODS

It is usually impossible to prevent some air getting into your baby's tummy along with the feed, so you may want to wind her, to release this air.

There are various ways of winding a baby, see suggestions below. Generally, air is released when you straighten the escape route vertically:

- hold your baby upright on your lap in a sitting position. Cup her chin in your hand, and gently stroke her back
- hold your baby high up on your shoulder, so that her tummy is resting on the top of your chest. Walking to and fro, patting her back gently often brings up wind
- sit down and lay your baby face down over your lap with one of your knees higher than the other, so that her head is uppermost. Gently rub her back.

5 If your baby seems very discontented, try bringing up her wind, using any of the methods suggested on the left.

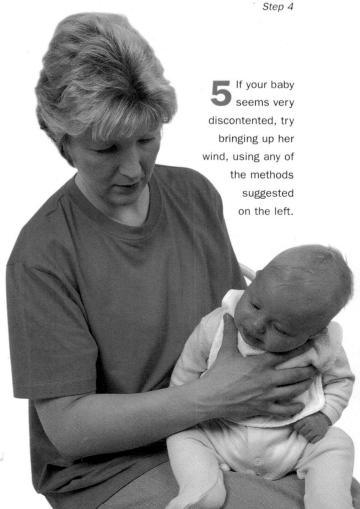

MIXING BREAST AND BOTTLE

More and more women are now choosing mixed feeding, which means using a flexible combination of breast milk and artificial milk for their baby.

A growing number of women are now returning to work before they are ready to give up breastfeeding. Apart from the health benefits, many want to breastfeed as a way of keeping close and maintaining that unique bond with their baby that no one else can replicate. Breastfeeding at the beginning and end of a working day can be particularly pleasurable for both mother and baby.

Others mix breast and bottle because it's also becoming popular to share the enjoyment of feeding with a partner, whilst still continuing to breastfeed.

FLEXIBILITY

If you are returning to work and want to carry on breastfeeding, you can express your milk, and store it, so that your baby receives only breast milk. Alternatively, you can breastfeed at home, and your child's carer can give formula milk in your absence.

Because breastfeeding works by adjusting its production according to the demand made, this means that you can be flexible about how much breast milk and how much formula milk you plan to give your baby.

When you feed your baby a bottle of formula milk, your milk supply responds to the reduction in demand by producing less milk. You may, for example, want to breastfeed for the first two feeds of the day, then offer formula milk for the mid-day feeds, finishing up by breastfeeding your baby yourself during the evening. Within days, you will find that your milk supply adapts to the changes.

Note: Give your body time to adjust to these changes, though. Don't drop more than one feed every three to four days.

FIRST THINGS FIRST

Before embarking on a routine of mixed feeding, it is important to get your milk supply established. During the first four to six weeks, the supply may be erratic, responding to a baby who has little or no routine as yet. If you try to experiment with mixed feeding before your breast milk has established itself, you may encounter more problems keeping the supply stable. It is far better to concentrate on building up an abundant milk supply in the early weeks, and to leave the fine tuning of mixed feeding until later.

Not too early, not too late: when, then?

'I introduced a bottle at four weeks and from then on, Lydia took both breast and bottle. Neil fed her with the bottle, and I expressed milk.'

'At six weeks, I tried – and failed. It was too late by then.'

If you are going to introduce bottle-feeding to run alongside breastfeeding, your baby needs to be able to alternate smoothly between the different textures, smells and techniques of sucking that come with breast and bottle. This is expecting a lot of a newborn and it does depend on the character of the individual child.

Introduce a bottle too early, and the baby may find feeding from the bottle preferable to waiting for the let down of milk from the breast. Introduce a bottle too late, and you'll find the baby is used to the breast and will not tolerate any substitute.

The right time can seem a bit of a lottery, but most mothers introduce a bottle between three and six weeks. By this time feeding is more or less established, yet there is still some flexibility about feeding methods.

If you are introducing a bottle in the early weeks simply in order to acclimatise your baby to the methods of bottle-feeding, don't offer it more than once or twice a week. You can offer either water, formula milk, or expressed breast milk at this stage, but remember, offering anything other than breast milk is likely to result in an equivalent drop in your supply.

BOOSTING YOUR MILK SUPPLY

Your milk supply may drop, particularly when you start the change from exclusive breastfeeding to mixed feeding. This may be because your baby starts to prefer feeding from a bottle and begins to breastfeed less. The supply can also drop if you return to work and start rushing around a lot more than before, not taking good care of your nutritional needs.

If you feel that your milk supply is running down, boost it by breastfeeding more often and making sure that you are eating, drinking and resting properly. Offer both breasts at each feed and express any remaining milk after a feed. Also try resting with your baby – take her to bed with you and let her feed whenever she wants to. Just as, when you feed less, you make less milk, so feeding more will make more milk for you. You should find that within a day or so, your milk supply has increased again.

COLIC

Colic is something that all parents dread. It's also something that's rather misunderstood. Even medical professionals disagree about what it is, some maintaining that it's caused by digestive problems, others saying that there's no hard evidence for this being the case. Parents, though, know that there is a condition, which many call colic, that affects some babies between approximately three weeks and three months of age. It's characterised by persistent, often frantic, crying, frequently accompanied by the baby drawing her knees up to her tummy, as if in pain, and going red in the face. It occurs mostly in the evening (usually every evening), and may go on for several hours. Nothing you try seems to stop the crying.

Unfortunately, there's no one proven cure for colic. If your baby suffers from it, there is little you can do other than wait for it to pass. It will pass, often as suddenly as it began, though that can be small consolation when you're going through it. If it makes you feel better to do something, you can try walking around with her held in an upright position, gently rubbing her tummy or giving her some gripe water. Tell your health visitor about the problem, too, because she will be able to help.

Some parents whose babies have suffered from colic have had them treated by a cranial osteopath. Many of them have reported that the osteopath's gentle manipulation of their baby's skull has improved the colic. It might be worth a try, but choose a qualified practitioner.

EXPRESSING BREAST MILK

There are times when it's useful to be able to express breast milk: for example, if your breasts are very full and your baby can't latch on, you are returning to work or you want to go out for the evening, or if your baby is in special care.

You can express milk either by hand, or with a breast pump. Whichever method you prefer, it may take time for you to become proficient. For some, the mechanical nature of a pump is off-putting. For others, hand expressing is tricky. You'll soon find out which method works best for you.

TRIGGERING THE LET DOWN

First of all, you have to 'trigger' your let down reflex. Take a few deep breaths, sigh out and let the tension flow out of you. Be patient and confident and know that it will happen. Warmth and relaxation will help, but it may take a little while initially. Thinking about your baby (perhaps having a photograph of her to look at if you are away from her) can help.

> ### GOOD TIMES TO EXPRESS MILK
> • when you are relaxed
> • after your baby has fed: either immediately, or an hour or so later
> • after your baby's first feed of the day.

As you feel happier with expressing milk, you will find that you gain confidence and it gets easier and easier.

One of the best times to express is after an early morning feed. Your body has been resting overnight, which is when it is best at making milk and very often your supply is more abundant than your baby might need.

If you opt for expressing straight after one of your baby's feeds, your baby will have stimulated the let down reflex, so you won't be starting from cold. Another way is to use a one-hand pump, so that you can feed the baby from one breast while expressing from the other. This may take some practice before it works well.

Another thing about the let down reflex is that it doesn't only appear at the very beginning of the feed, but kicks in spasmodically throughout. This means that if you happen to be expressing and feel that the milk is running out, you may find that if you keep going a little longer, there will be another surge of milk. It's important, though, to stop expressing if you start to feel sore.

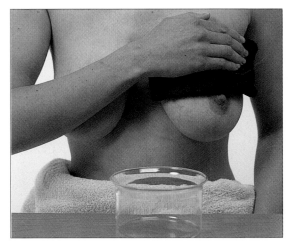

1 Before starting to express, warm your breast with a flannel or cloth. This will help to trigger the let down reflex and encourage the milk to flow.

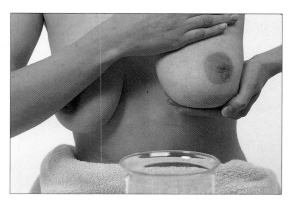

2 Holding your breast gently with one hand, move all around it with the other, massaging from the outer edge of the breast towards the nipple.

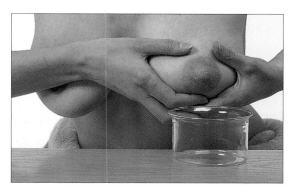

3 Position your hand behind the areola and start to squeeze gently. Try pushing in towards your rib cage before rolling your fingers inwards.

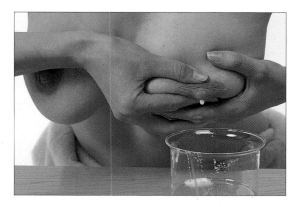

4 As you start to squeeze, milk will come out of your breast. Move your hand around your breast to remove milk from all the ducts.

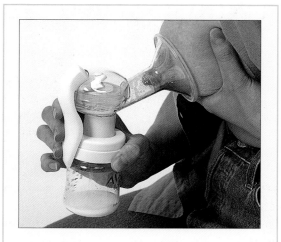

USING A BREAST PUMP

You can buy different types of breast pumps: manual, battery and electric. Some pumps have soft inner flanges which gently massage the area around the nipple, encouraging the let down reflex.

The same principles apply to using a pump as to hand expressing: equipment must be sterile, use relaxation and warmth to stimulate the let down, and persevere.

EXPRESSING AT WORK

If conditions at work make it difficult to express milk, remember that under existing health and safety laws, employers have legal obligations to provide facilities for mothers and to enable them to express and store milk if they wish. If you work in the public sector, you will also be covered by the European Pregnant Worker's Directive which states that if a mother's working conditions or hours affect her breastfeeding, the employer must change them or give her alternative work.

The Maternity Alliance can help with this; find their address on page 250.

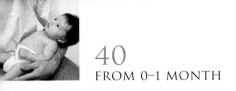
SLEEP AND THE NEW PARENT

There are few parents who can say that they get enough sleep when their new baby is born.

Nobody can tell you how your baby will sleep, but you can be pretty sure that she won't be sleeping through the night, and you are unlikely to find that she follows a regular pattern for a number of weeks. As your baby grows, she will sleep for longer periods of time.

It is important to grasp any sleep opportunities with both hands. For the first week or two, it really can pay off if you can drop everything, forget the housework and rest when your baby rests. If you can't bear the thought of sleeping throughout her sleep, why not lie down or rest in a chair for half an hour, with your alarm clock set? This short nap can act as a valuable refresher.

'If she woke in the night, it could take three hours to get her off again.'

SLEEP AND THE NEW BABY

Your newborn baby is likely to sleep wherever she is put, regardless of what is going on around her. However, there may be times when she needs a little help dropping off. Try the following:

• Movement

Most babies like to be rocked or swayed and it often lulls them into sleep. You can cuddle your baby and rock from side to side with her in your arms, or you can put her in a sling, so you can get on with what you are doing while she's tucked up next to you. You will soon learn which way your baby prefers to be held, and how she responds to different movements.

A walk outside with the baby in her pram often brings sleep, as does taking her out in the car. The rhythmical movement and drone of the engine can bring distraction, which may be all that is needed for her to drift into sleep. Make sure you drive or walk for long enough to let her get into a deep sleep before you come home (but unfortunately there are no guarantees that she'll stay sleeping for long once you're back!).

• Comfort

Like all of us, your baby needs to feel safe and secure before she falls asleep. Cuddling your baby, stroking her and talking in a gentle, calm voice will all help to settle her.

Your baby should feel warm, but not hot. Some babies feel more secure if they are wrapped up snugly, but others throw their covers off. See which she prefers.

Babies get a great deal of pleasure out of sucking, so whether you prefer to give breast, bottle or a dummy, your baby should find this reassuring. At this very early stage, don't worry if she falls asleep on the breast or bottle. It would be virtually impossible to stop her.

• Noise

You might imagine that noise wakes babies up, but often it can be the distraction that helps them to sleep.

Try putting the vacuum cleaner or a hairdryer on for a few minutes. This 'white noise' can often do the trick. Some mothers even use a washing machine on a fast spin cycle or a radio that's not quite properly tuned into a station!

You could sing to your baby, or talk to her quietly, telling her a story, or even put some music on. Whether these are distractions, moving the baby on from crying, or whether they are genuinely calming is not really known. But they often do the trick.

WHERE YOUR BABY SLEEPS

Newborn babies sleep for about 60% of their day, that is, about 14 to 18 hours in 24. You may prefer to have her close by you for her long sleeps during the daytime so that you can keep an eye on her, at first. Since noise is unlikely to disturb her, there is no need to put her in a separate room. In fact, as has been said, she may well feel more secure if she hears noises around her, just as she did in the womb.

If you live on more than one floor, have somewhere for the baby to sleep on every level, particularly if you have had a caesarean section and shouldn't be carrying your baby around.

Many parents like having their baby in their own bedroom, as this means they can be close when the baby wakes. Others prefer the baby to have a separate bedroom from day one. You will find your own preference when the time comes.

'We relied on driving Alice round in the car to get her off to sleep and then she could be lifted out without waking.'

Remember that if your baby is out of earshot, you should use a baby listener, and if you have pets, make sure that they cannot get into the baby's cot. It goes without saying that your baby should always be in a smoke-free atmosphere.

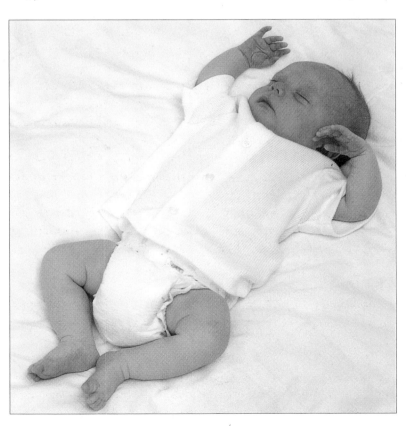

EACH BABY IS DIFFERENT

You will find out your baby's preferences by experimenting. Each baby is different and won't conform to a 'type'. Take your time just getting to know her as she is, and don't worry if she is different from the baby next door – you're probably very different from the mother next door!

You will probably find that every day is different too, and you may find the disruption hard to cope with. Gradually, a routine will form and you'll feel less overwhelmed. Don't panic!

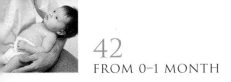
STEP BY STEP MAKING UP A COT

The most important thing about making up a cot for your baby is doing it in such a way that he's as safe as possible when he's in it.

Here's how to ensure that your baby won't wriggle right down under the covers and get overheated in his cot.

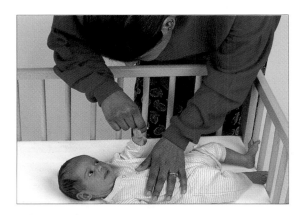

1 Place your baby in the cot so that his feet are a few centimetres away from the end of the cot (think 'feet to foot' – that is, have the baby's feet at the foot of the cot). Like that, he can't wriggle down the cot in his sleep and end up with the covers over his head. Put him on his back or side, not his front.

2 Lay the top sheet over your baby so that it comes up to his shoulders and tuck it under the mattress at the sides and the bottom. You may need to fold the sheet in half so that it's not too big. Tuck it in so that it's snug, but not too restricting. In hot weather, a sheet may be all that your baby needs.

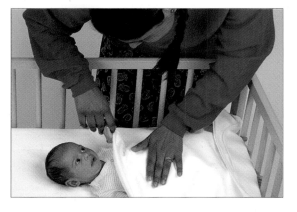

3 Lay the blanket over the sheet, so that it too comes up to your baby's shoulders, and tuck it in, though not so tightly that he can't kick it off if he gets too hot. You'll probably need to fold it in half.

4 If your house is centrally heated, two or three layers of blanket (a single folded blanket equals two layers) will be enough. If it isn't, you may need a fourth layer. You can remove or add a layer if your baby seems to be too hot or too cold.

BEDDING FOR YOUR BABY'S COT

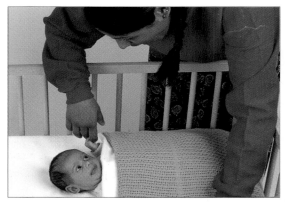

- a cotton sheet to put over the mattress, plus any spares you want for when it's being washed
- a cotton top sheet, plus spares

• one or two cotton cellular blankets, plus spares. Using cotton blankets reduces the possibility of your baby overheating. Don't use a duvet for a baby under a year. Sheepskins and baby nests can also make a baby too hot and are best avoided for sleeping

• don't use pillows or a cot bumper. Babies need to lose heat from the top of their heads while they sleep, so don't put anything behind your baby's head that could restrict this heat loss. This includes cuddly toys. The cot may look rather bare, but it will be safer for your baby that way

• use a firm mattress and keep it flat, dry and well aired. Avoid using any mattress that seems lumpy or soft, as some second-hand ones can be. The claim that some types of mattress give off a toxic gas that can cause cot death has been shown by recent research to be unlikely to be true. Make sure that the mattress is large enough for the cot, with not more than a 4cm space anywhere around the edge.

MOSES BASKET OR CARRYCOT

New babies may not like being put in a cot because it makes them feel exposed and insecure. For the first few months, they may feel more comfortable sleeping in a Moses basket or crib or carrycot. If you decide to use one of these, make it up in the same way as shown here, using the same kind of bedding. Make sure that it isn't left in a draught or near a fire or radiator when your baby is in it. It's also safer not to leave it on a raised surface – other than a stand or chassis designed specifically for it. If you have a cat, use a cat net.

When the time comes for your baby to move into a cot, you can make the transition easier by putting him in his Moses basket or carrycot inside the cot for a while to help him to get used to the cot gradually.

COT DEATH

Although cot death, or sudden infant death syndrome, is rare, it's something that all parents worry about – to the extent that the first time your baby sleeps through the night, you'll probably find that you're up several times to check that he's still breathing.

The cause of cot death is unknown – it may be due to a combination of factors affecting a baby at a time when he's particularly vulnerable to them, though we don't know exactly what these factors are. We do know, though, that taking the following steps can help minimise the risk of it happening:

• Put your baby on his back to sleep, not on his front or side.

• Position your baby in his cot as shown here ('feet to foot').

• Take care that your baby doesn't overheat. Use cotton sheets and blankets, never pillows or a duvet. Don't leave him to sleep near a radiator or fire, or in direct sunlight. Aim to keep the room temperature at around 18°C (although in the first few days it should ideally be slightly higher than this).

• Don't smoke near your baby and don't let anyone smoke inside the house at all.

• Breastfeeding is best for babies, though the research evidence on whether it offers any kind of specific protection against cot death is currently mixed.

• The current research evidence on whether there is any link between co-sleeping (see page 95) and cot death is also mixed. The Foundation for the Study of Infant Death at present recommends that your baby sleeps in a cot beside your bed, rather than in your bed, until he is at least six months old.

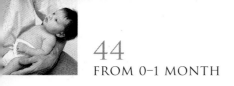

COMFORTING A CRYING BABY

Babies cry. It's their way of communicating to you that they want something. Parents (and others) want babies to stop crying. That's nature's way of making sure that babies' needs are met.

There's no noise quite so distressing as the sound of your own baby crying. Unfortunately, soothing your crying baby isn't always easy, because it's so hard to tell, especially at first, exactly what it is that she wants. So you may have to use guesswork to find it out. Sometimes you manage to get there straight away and everyone's happy. Sometimes you don't, and they're not.

WHY YOUR BABY MIGHT BE CRYING

If your baby's crying, the first obvious cause to eliminate is hunger. If she's hungry, nothing that you can do apart from feed her will comfort her. If she's just had a feed, she may be crying because she has wind. Or she may need her nappy changing.

If neither top nor bottom ends seem to be in need of attention, your baby may be crying because she's too hot or too cold. Or she may just want a cuddle. Some babies seem only to be happy when they're being held (in countries where babies are carried next to their mothers' bodies most of the time, they rarely cry). If your baby wants to be held a lot, you may find a sling invaluable. It will allow you both to give her the physical contact she wants and to get on with other things that you need to do.

If you can't carry her, try wrapping her in a blanket or towel or swaddling her instead, to make her feel as if she's being held (see page 20). Swaddling can also help calm a baby who's crying because she's become distressed by the 'wide open space' feeling that comes with being undressed or bathed.

Babies also sometimes cry because they're overstimulated or tired, and they need to be left alone to rest or to go to sleep.

Sometimes you can eliminate all these causes, and your baby still cries. 'Unless he's actually feeding, Max just screams all the time,' says Caroline. 'He seems to be frustrated about something, but I don't know what.' Some babies just don't seem to like being babies – they want to be doing things but they're not yet able to, and they cry with frustration. Others find it hard to cope with life outside the womb – the new sensations, such as hunger and tiredness, and different levels of stimulation, such as loud noises and bright lights, overwhelm them.

SOOTHING YOUR BABY

Parents who can't identify why their baby is crying can be extremely inventive in coming up with ways to soothe her. If you need to, you'll find your own individual solution, probably after a process of trial and error. Solutions that have worked for other parents include:

• rocking her in your arms or in a bouncing cradle

• taking her for a walk in her pram or buggy (if it's the middle of the night, push her round the garden or even indoors)

• putting her in her car seat and taking her for

a drive, though she may start to cry again when you take her out of the car

• playing a womb music tape (look for one in the small ads at the back of a baby magazine)

• playing any kind of soothing music, especially something you find relaxing

• singing to her

• putting her near a domestic appliance that makes a humming noise – like a vacuum cleaner or a washing machine. (Don't put her cradle on top of the washing machine, in case of falls.)

• letting her suck on your little finger (make sure it's clean and the nail is short) or helping her to suck her own hand. Some parents give their baby a dummy. There are disadvantages to dummies but some parents find that if it stops the crying, they can live with the disadvantages

• trying to relax yourself, although it can be remarkably difficult with a crying baby. It may be that if you're feeling too tense,

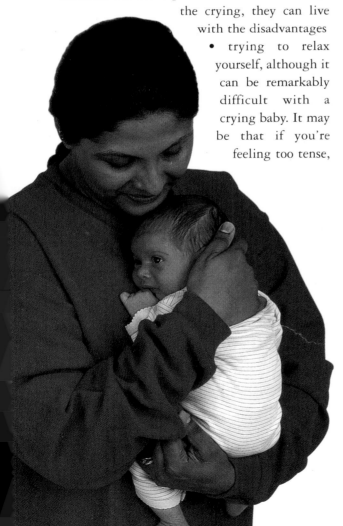

you're transmitting tension to your baby and making the crying worse.

If you find it impossible to soothe your baby, she could be ill. Contact your doctor if you have any reason to think that she might be.

COPING WITH A CRYING BABY

Having a baby who seems to cry all the time can be a soul-destroying experience. You want so much to make her happy, but you just don't seem to be able to. It doesn't help matters that the time babies cry the most – during the first three months – is also the time when you may be feeling your least confident about being a parent. If you can, try and hang on to the thought that the crying phase will pass (it will).

Almost all parents at some point find that their baby's crying becomes too much. If this happens to you, and you feel you just can't cope any more, put your baby gently in a safe place and go into another room for a few minutes. Then try one or more of the following:

• close your eyes and take several deep breaths. Some people also find it helps to imagine themselves in a peaceful place

• count to ten (or 100, if you're very wound up)

• turn on the radio or television so that you can't hear the baby crying

• shout at the wall (it's better than shouting at the baby) or sing loudly

• punch, shake or throw a pillow

• phone a friend and let your feelings out.

When you feel calmer, go back to your baby and give her a cuddle.

These are short-term solutions. If you find you're getting stressed every day because of your baby's crying, see if you can arrange for someone else to look after the baby for a couple of hours so you can have a break. If you're getting desperate, talk to your health visitor or GP.

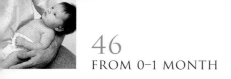
CHOOSING EQUIPMENT

Buying equipment for your baby can be fun, but it can also be bewildering. With such a huge range of things on offer in the baby shops, it's not always easy to know what you really need.

When you buy equipment for your baby, it can be difficult to be sure that you're spending your money wisely. There's such an array of different makes and styles to choose from. No wonder a lot of parents-to-be are like Jessica and Paul: 'We spent two and a half hours looking at prams and ended up coming out of the shop with some cotton wool and breast pads.'

WHEN TO BUY WHAT

Parents-to-be have different ideas about the timing of buying equipment. 'I don't want to buy much for the baby before it's born, because it seems like tempting fate,' says Louise.

Sally has taken a different approach: 'We've bought everything we think we're going to need because we don't expect to have much time for shopping once the baby's arrived'.

Richard and Penny are hedging their bets: 'We want to spread the expense, so we've bought a few things now, and we'll get others as we find we need them'.

IN THE EARLY MONTHS YOU NEED

- nappies and clothing
- changing mat
- towels and toiletries
- muslin squares
- breastfeeding bras or bottles etc.
- Moses basket or carrycot or crib for sleeping in, plus mattress and bedding

- baby bath
- sling
- car seat
- pram or lie-back buggy
- bouncing cradle or baby rocker
- baby listener

IN LATER MONTHS YOU NEED

- cot, plus mattress and bedding
- perhaps a baby bouncer
- high chair
- beakers, bowls, spoons
- backpack
- 'umbrella' buggy

BABY ON A BUDGET

Many first-time parents-to-be are like David. 'I'm terrified about money. Our income is about to go down and our expenditure is shooting up.'

If your budget is tight, there are ways in which you can equip your baby for less.
- Look in the classified ads section of your local paper for items that you want
- Look out for nearly new sales, such as those organised by your local NCT branch
- Go to car boot sales
- Buy as much as you can in the sales
- Encourage friends to lend or pass something on to you!

Where baby equipment is concerned, second-hand doesn't necessarily mean second best. But if you are buying things second-hand, or being given or lent them, always check them from a safety point of view.

CAR SEATS

If you drive, your baby will need a car seat. Rear-facing car seats are safer for small babies than forward-facing ones, and are safer used on the back seat, rather than the front. (Never use a rear-facing seat on the front seat of a car with a passenger airbag.) Make sure that the harness will hold your baby securely and can be easily adjusted. Other things that you might like to look for include carrying handles and removable washable covers, and how padded the seat is. And always make sure that the seat you choose conforms to government safety standards.

If you can, try the seat out in your car (or cars if you have more than one) to check that it fits before you buy it. If you can't do this, make sure that you can take the seat back if it doesn't fit.

Some garages will check the fit of a seat in your car for you. Your local council's Road Safety Department should be able to tell you the nearest garage offering this service.

Some parents choose to buy a baby seat, which lasts till their baby is around nine months, then a child seat, which lasts till he's around four. Others choose to buy a combined baby/child seat, which will take their baby from birth to four. The combined seat tends to work out cheaper in the long run – though may be more expensive initially – but it can be awkward to lift in and out of the car.

PRAMS AND BUGGIES

For many parents, choosing which pram or buggy to buy can be one of the hardest purchasing decisions they have to make. Should it be a traditional pram? A lightweight buggy?

A pram that converts to a pushchair? One that can be forward- or rear-facing? One with a detachable carrycot or an attachable car seat? As well as taking your budget into account, it can help to think in advance about how you're going to use the pram or buggy. Do you need something that will fold easily so that you can take it on a bus or put it in the boot of a car? Do you walk everywhere so need something large and solid? Will you have to carry it up stairs? Do you want to be able to carry a lot of shopping on it? Do you want to use it till your baby is three or four years of age, or will you then switch to something different, like an 'umbrella' buggy, when he's older? Have you got room for it in your house?

'We bought a perfectly good buggy at a car boot sale for a fraction of the price brand new.'

When your baby is new, you'll need a pram or buggy in which he can lie flat. Once he has developed head and neck control, which comes at about four months, he can be sat in a more upright position. In either case, he'll be safest if he's secured with a five-point harness. If your pram or buggy doesn't come with one, you can buy one separately.

Other factors that you might want to take into account include whether the height of the handle is comfortable for you, and how manoeuvrable the pram or pushchair is.

If you opt for a buggy rather than a pram, you'll need rain covers, a sun canopy and maybe a 'cosytoes', so don't forget to allow for these in your cost calculations. Check that the buggy will fold easily with these attached, or you'll be endlessly dismantling the whole thing to put them on and take them off.

As with car seats, make sure that any model you buy conforms to British or European safety standards.

STEP BY STEP
PUTTING ON A SLING

The key to putting on a sling without running the risk of your baby falling out is to get the baby securely into it, on a firm surface, before you put the sling onto yourself.

'It was like being in one of those game shows where you have to perform some impossible task against the clock. Except on the game shows, they don't have to worry about dropping their baby.' That was how Ali felt about trying to put a sling on at first. 'I thought I'd never get the hang of it, although I have to say now I find it quite easy.' Here's how to do it:

1 Lay the sling on a flat surface with the opening facing upwards and the straps out to the side.

2 Position your baby on her back in the sling's opening.

3 Gently guide your baby's legs into the leg holes if the sling has them, and fasten any straps around her tummy.

4 Once she's securely in the sling, slide one hand under her bottom, outside the sling, and the other behind her head, and lift her towards you, supporting her head.

5 Let your baby rest against your body with her head on your chest. Support her bottom with one hand, and put one of the shoulder straps over your shoulder with other hand. You may find it easier to do this if you lean back slightly. Do the same with the

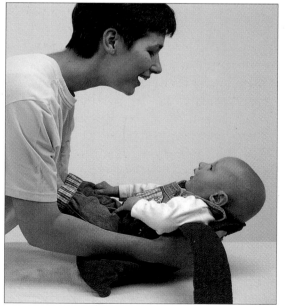

Step 2

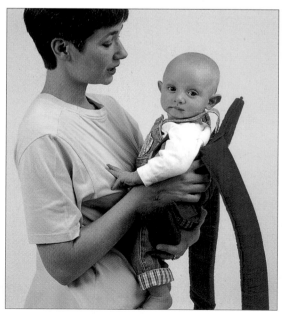

Step 4

other strap (you may need to switch hands). If you have the straps adjusted so that your baby is held against your chest rather than your tummy, you'll put less of a strain on your back when you're carrying her.

6 Fasten the straps around your middle and tie them up in a big bow.

Alternatively, get someone else to help you.

CHOOSING A SLING

There are lots of different slings on the market but most of them are of one of two types. The first, sometimes called a front carrier, has straps which go over your shoulders and round your waist. It holds your baby in an upright position (as shown below).

The second type is worn across one shoulder, like a sash. It forms a sort of hammock, in which your baby either lies or sits.

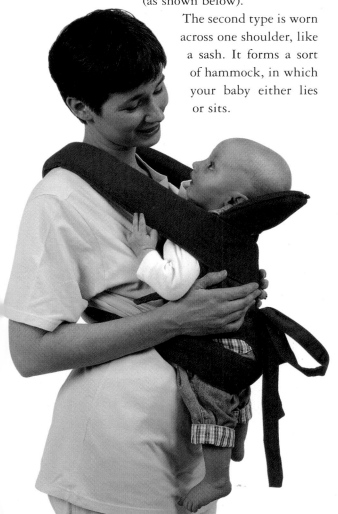

CARRY ME!

If you put your finger in the palm of a new baby's hand, he will grasp it tightly. Although, unlike our early ancestors from whom this reflex is inherited, babies no longer need to be able to cling on to the hair on their mothers' bodies, they still have a strong need to be carried – something that we in our modern western society of buggies, car seats and bouncy chairs sometimes forget.

Babies are often at their most content when they're being held. Carrying your baby provides him with warmth and security, as well as giving him the reassurance of hearing the familiar sound of your heartbeat and feeling your familiar movements. It also allows him to be involved in what you're doing – even though it generally makes it more difficult to do it.

Some babies are only content when they're being held. They cry until they're picked up, and they cry again if they're put down. Swaddling them will sometimes fool them into thinking they're being held, but more often than not only physical contact will do. Parents develop their own strategies for handling a baby like this. Many choose to do what parents have done for centuries the world over, and get a sling, so that they can give their baby the comfort of being carried while keeping their hands free to do other things.

Carrying your baby for what can seem like hours on end can undoubtedly be tiring. But if it makes your baby more content and relaxed, you're likely to feel content and relaxed too; and at least you'll be using your energy in a positive way.

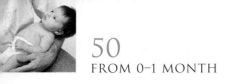

STEP BY STEP
BATHING YOUR BABY

Small babies don't get very dirty, and if baths are unpopular, you can keep them to a minimum at first – once or twice a week is fine – and make do with daily topping and tailing instead.

Your new baby may seem very fragile, you may not be feeling confident about handling her, and to top it all she screams blue murder when you take her clothes off. No wonder the prospect of bathing her doesn't seem very appealing at first! Don't worry – eventually the point will come when you give her a bath and find that she actually enjoys it, and you will too!

1 Make sure the room is warm – your baby will cry if she's cold. Aim for 21°C or above.

2 Get everything that you need to hand before you get your baby ready (see facing page).

3 Fill the bath with water to a depth of about 10cm. Put cold water in first, then add the hot. You can check the temperature of the water by dipping your elbow into it (it should feel warm) or with a special baby bath thermometer.

4 Undress your baby down to her nappy, talking to her to help keep her calm.

5 Wrap her in a towel – you can do this in the same way as if you were swaddling her (see page 20). If her arms are wrapped under the towel, you won't have to cope with them flailing around.

6 Wash her face with cotton wool dipped in cooled boiled water.

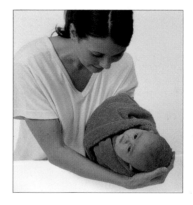

7 Supporting her back along your arm and her head in your hand, hold her head over the side of the bath. Hold her securely but gently against your side, with her head tipped down slightly so that water won't run into her eyes. Using your hand, or a jug, or a sponge, pour some of the bathwater over her head. For tiny babies, rinsing their hair is usually enough to keep it clean, though if your baby has a lot of hair, you might want to use a little shampoo. If you do use shampoo, rinse it off with the bathwater, then rinse again with some clean water.

8 Pat her head dry with a separate towel, trying not to cover her face, which may make her panic.

9 Put her on a changing mat, unwrap the towel, take her nappy off and clean her bottom.

10 Pick her up and, cradling her with your arm behind her shoulders and your hand under her arm to support her head, and with your other hand supporting her bottom, lower her into the water. Talking to her as you do so will help to reassure her.

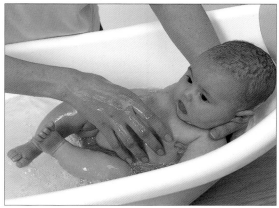

Step 11

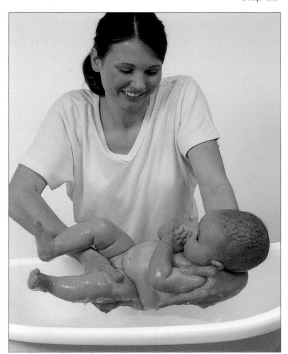

Step 12

12 Lift her out holding her as you did when you put her in (she'll be slippery now) and wrap her snugly in a towel, pulling it round her head. You can dry her either by cuddling her on your lap or by laying her on a changing mat and patting her dry. Check that all the creases in her skin are dry before putting on her clean nappy and clothes.

WHAT YOU NEED FOR BATHING

• a baby bath or a large washing-up bowl which you can stand on a firm surface. Some baby baths fit over an ordinary bath, making them easy to fill and empty. You can also use the sink too, but wrap a flannel or towel around the taps in case your baby bumps against them
• one or two warm towels and a changing mat
• clean nappy and clean clothes to put on afterwards. Nappy-changing equipment
• cooled boiled water and cotton wool for washing your baby's face
• if you're going to wash your baby's hair with shampoo, a jug of clean warm water for rinsing
• mild bath liquid or soap and mild shampoo if you want to use these. Talcum powder, though it smells lovely, is best avoided as your baby could breathe it in and harm her lungs.

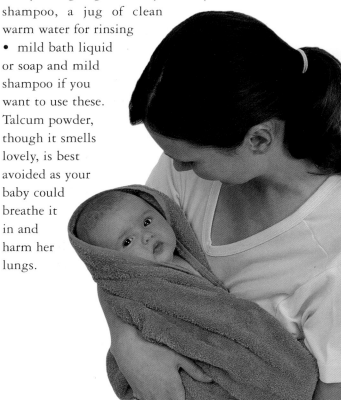

11 Once she's used to this, you can take away the hand supporting her bottom, but keep hold of her arm so that her head and shoulders stay supported. Use your other hand to gently swish the water over her and rub her body clean. Some parents feel more confident putting their baby on a bath support. Don't leave her in the bath for more than a couple of minutes.

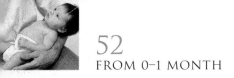
STEP BY STEP
TOPPING AND TAILING

Although your baby doesn't need to be bathed every day, he does need his top and bottom ends to be kept clean. Thankfully, most babies don't seem to object to daily 'topping and tailing' and many of them rather enjoy it.

What you need for topping and tailing your baby: • a changing mat • a clean nappy (and clean clothes if you're going to change them) • a bowl of cooled boiled water • cotton wool or clean flannel • a towel • a bin to put the used nappy and used cotton wool in.

1 Lay your baby on his back on a changing mat covered with a towel or terry nappy, or sit him on your lap. You might find the 'topping' easier if you wrap him in a towel to restrain waving arms. There's no need to undress him, unless you want to.

2 Wipe one eye with a piece of cotton wool moistened with cooled boiled water. Wipe from the inside corner of the eye outwards. Then wipe the other eye using a fresh piece of cotton wool.

3 Wipe over his ears (including behind them) with damp cotton wool, using a fresh piece for each ear. Wipe over his face, neck and under his chin with another piece of damp cotton wool or a damp flannel.

4 Pat him dry with a small soft towel, making sure that there's no dampness in the creases.

5 Wipe his hands and dry them.

6 Change his nappy (see page 56) and put on his clean clothes if you're changing them.

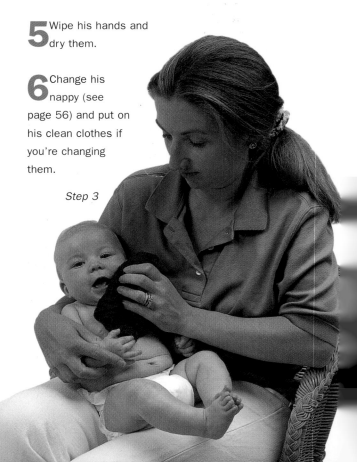

Step 3

Step 2

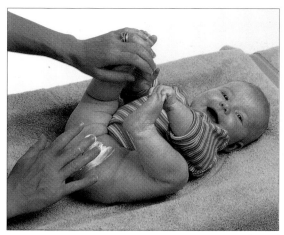

Step 6

HAIR CARE

There's no need to wash your baby's hair – if he has any – every day. Wiping over it with a damp flannel will remove any dribble or regurgitated milk or anything else that has got into it.

Cradle cap

This is an extremely common condition characterised by yellow brown scales forming on the baby's scalp. It's quite harmless and the only reason for doing anything about it is that it doesn't look very nice.

If your baby has cradle cap and you want to try and get rid of it, you can rub some baby oil into his scalp and leave it overnight – or longer. This may loosen the scales, which may then come off when you wash his hair. You may need to try this several times before it works, and it doesn't always succeed. Combing can help remove the scales, though don't be tempted to pick them off with your fingernails – that can make the condition worse. Cradle cap usually clears up in a few weeks, but in some cases it can last for months.

Rarely, cradle cap can extend to form a rash over your baby's face and neck. If this happens, consult your doctor.

KEEPING THE TRICKY BITS CLEAN

- **Nails**

Babies' fingernails need to be kept short, as babies tend to hold their hands near their faces and can scratch themselves.

Some parents find that the easiest way to cut their baby's nails is simply to nibble them off themselves, perhaps after – or even during – a feed when they have their baby in their arms and he's relaxed. Others find this difficult and prefer to use round-ended scissors or baby nail clippers. It can be difficult to hold the baby and use scissors at the same time, so lay your baby down, or wait till he's asleep. Toenails are less of a scratching hazard but still need to be trimmed. If you try after a bath, they will be softer and easier to cut.

- **Ears and nose**

Your baby's ears and nose are self-cleaning and there's no need ever to put anything inside them to clean them. Just clean gently round the openings with damp cotton wool.

- **Cord**

The cord stump is best left alone. There's no need to wash it, though you can clean the skin around it if necessary. Getting it wet in the bath won't harm it, though make sure you dry it carefully afterwards. If you think it looks sticky or irritated, ask your midwife to check it. Don't worry if it turns black – that's normal. The stump usually drops off in 7–10 days.

- **Genitals**

A good principle to apply is wash only what you can see. Don't try and clean inside a girl's vulva, or pull back a boy's foreskin to clean under it. These parts can clean themselves better than you can, and if you try, you may cause some damage.

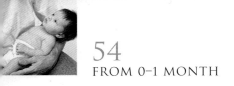

NAPPY CHOICES

With almost 6,000 nappy changes to get through until your baby is potty-trained, you need to be using a type of nappy that suits you and the baby.

For some parents, their circumstances or their convictions make it easy for them to choose what nappies to use. For others, it's a matter of weighing up the pros and cons of the options, and making a decision on balance.

Broadly speaking, the decision comes down to whether to use disposables or washables.

DISPOSABLES

Your friend may swear by a particular brand of disposable nappy; *Which?* may recommend something else. But what suits one baby doesn't necessarily suit another, so you may need to try different kinds until you find one that's right for your baby.

Reasons for disposables
- easy to use – wherever you are
- very absorbent so less likely to leak – but don't let yourself be tempted to leave your baby in the same nappy for several hours because it seems to be dry
- easily obtainable from supermarkets, chemists, 24-hour garages (useful if you run out at night). Some shops will deliver in bulk, which saves lugging large quantities of nappies home with you. Don't buy too far ahead, though – babies grow very quickly

Reasons against
- cost
- fit. Babies come in all shapes and sizes and nappies don't. If your baby isn't a 'standard' size, you may have trouble finding a disposable that fits
- they contain a chemical gel that can irritate some babies' skin

Liz opted for disposables: 'As far as I'm concerned, washables use up far too much energy – mine.'

WASHABLE NAPPIES

If you decide to use washable nappies, the choice is between terry nappies – either the traditional square or the shaped type – and the newer fitted cloth nappies. The latter are shaped like a disposable, but are made of cloth. Some have a plastic outer cover, but with others you need to use plastic pants. If you choose terries, buy the best quality you can afford. You may need to put your baby in slightly larger clothes.

Reasons for washables
- made of natural fibres
- cost less. But don't forget to add the cost of laundering the nappies to the initial cost of buying them. And while terries are cheap compared to the cost of disposables, fitted nappies can be quite expensive
- square terries can be folded to suit your baby (see page 58 for ways to fold terries)

Reasons against
- you have to wash them
- they need to be soaked in sterilising solution (keep buckets out of reach of toddlers)

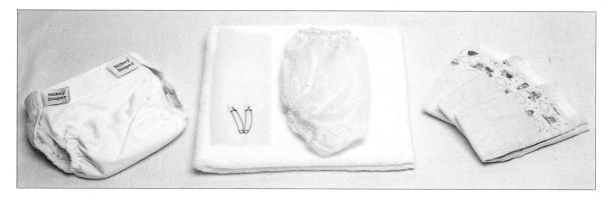

- getting them dry can be difficult
- although terry nappies are easy to find in shops that sell baby goods, other kinds of washable nappies may only be available by mail order (look in the small ads at the back of parenting magazines)
- you may have to use plastic pants
- they may be awkward to use away from home

  Juliet and Eric use terries: 'We're amazed how easy they are – it's just a question of being organised.'

NAPPIES AND THE ENVIRONMENT

Some parents are concerned about the environmental impact of nappies. Research on this has produced varied results, some studies finding that disposables are environmentally unfriendly and others finding that they're not. Most of these studies have been done either by disposable nappy manufacturers or by interest groups promoting washable nappies – you can no doubt predict which groups reached what conclusion.

- Disposable nappies produce more waste.
- Disposables are made from pulped wood and use up a lot of trees.
- Disposables are mostly disposed of in landfill sites, which are rapidly filling up. In areas where there is no landfill site, the waste has to be transported. (Though in some areas, it's

incinerated and that produces recoverable energy.)

- Washable nappies use electricity, which is produced by burning fossil fuels, which generates pollution.
- Washable nappies use detergent, which may pollute the water system.
- Washable nappies use up water.
- Growing cotton – from which most washable nappies are made – has an impact on the environment.
- Nappy services wash a lot of nappies together so use less electricity, water and detergent than individuals washing nappies at home.

WHAT YOU WILL NEED

Disposables

- nappies (6–8 a day on average: more in the early days, fewer in later months)
- nappy disposal bags
- wrap and seal bin – if you want to use one

Washable nappies

- around 20–24 nappies
- pins or fasteners for terries
- nappy liners
- plastic pants
- one or two plastic buckets with lids
- nappy sterilising powder or other sterilising substance.

STEP BY STEP
CHANGING A NAPPY

When your baby is very new, you'll find that you're changing her nappy about ten times a day. As your baby gets older, by which time you'll be a dab hand at it, you won't need to do it so often.

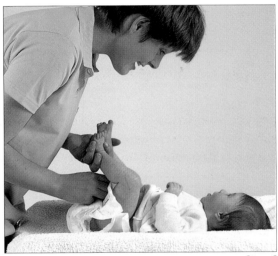

Step 3

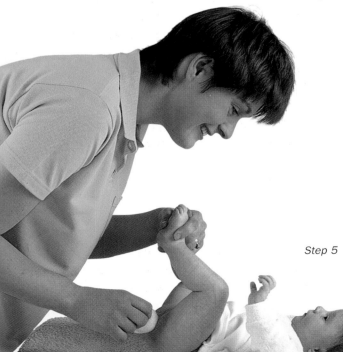

Step 5

Believe it or not, nappy-changing sessions can be fun. You'll probably find that instinctively you talk to your baby as you change her. This, together with smiling at her, and, when she's a little older, playing with her, can all make nappy-changing enjoyable, rather than just a chore.

To make it easier for yourself, try and get everything that you need together and within reach before you start – including somewhere to put the used nappy. It can be a good idea to have a change of clothes for the baby to hand too, just in case of accidents.

1 Put your baby on her back on a changing mat. The mat will feel less cold if you cover it with a towel or a terry or muslin nappy. It's better for your back if you can put her on a surface that you don't have to bend over too far to reach. If this is a raised surface, though, don't leave her unattended. She may not be able to roll over yet, but you never know when she's going to do so for the first time.

2 Undo the tabs or fasteners and lift the front of the nappy off. A boy may well pee at this point, so hold the nappy over his penis for a second or two.

3 If the nappy's dirty, wipe any poo off your baby's bottom using an unsoiled part of the nappy. Hold both her legs in one hand while you do this, otherwise she'll wave them around. If you put a finger between

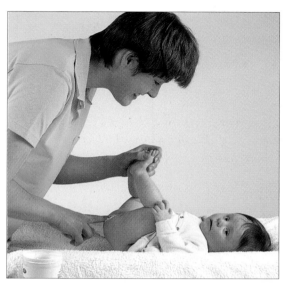

Step 7

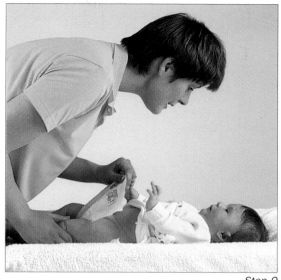

Step 9

her ankles, that will stop them from being pressed uncomfortably together.

4 When you've got the worst off, slide the nappy out from under her bottom, or fold it together and tuck it under her bottom while you clean her.

5 Still holding her legs, clean her bottom using cotton wool and warm water. You can also use baby lotion or oil, or baby wipes, but these can sometimes irritate babies' skin. Clean the whole area covered by the nappy – working from front to back for a girl – especially the creases in the skin. Pat her bottom dry with a soft tissue or towel.

6 If your baby likes being without a nappy, leave her for a few minutes to enjoy the air on her bottom – but don't leave her unattended. If you're using terries, assemble your nappy and liner.

7 You could apply a barrier cream, such as zinc and castor oil cream or Vaseline. Some disposable nappy manufacturers suggest a barrier cream is not necessary, either because the nappy has cream in it or because the nappy is designed to let air circulate.

8 Still holding her feet, slide the back of the clean nappy under her bottom so that the top of it is in line with her waist. If it's a disposable, don't undo the tabs yet.

9 Bring the front of the nappy between her legs (if your baby is a boy, point his penis towards his feet), and fasten the tabs. If they're adhesive tabs, as on a disposable, make sure you keep them free from cream or they won't stick properly. If you do get cream on them, you can try fastening the nappy with sticky tape. Slide a finger under the waistband to check it's not too tight.

10 Put her clothes back on, and you're all done (that is, until she immediately fills the new nappy and you have to start all over again).

11 Put your baby somewhere safe while you deal with the dirty nappy. If you're using a cloth nappy, sluice off any poo in the loo and put the nappy to soak in sterilising solution. If you're using a disposable, sluicing that in the loo before you put it in the bin will help reduce the amount of excrement that goes into landfill sites. Now wash your hands!

STEP BY STEP
FOLDING A TERRY NAPPY

Terry nappies come in two types, the traditional square nappy and the newer shaped nappy. The square nappies tend to be more widely available.

One of the advantages of square terries is that you can fold them to fit your baby, and adjust the fold as your baby grows.

For a small baby, the triple or 'origami' fold gives a small, neat shape. It can seem horribly complicated to do at first, but it becomes easy with practice.

1 On a flat surface, fold the nappy in half so that the fold is horizontal and facing towards you.

2 Lift up one of the loose corners and take it horizontally across to lie on top of the other loose corners (you'll now have a triangle of nappy resting on top of a square of nappy so that half of the square lies under half of the triangle – as in the picture).

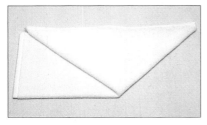

3 Turn the whole nappy the other way up. Hold the folds in place as you do so, otherwise you'll have to start all over again.

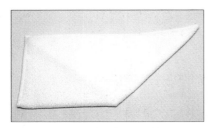

4 Lift up the two vertical edges and fold them in about a third of the way along the top horizontal edge.

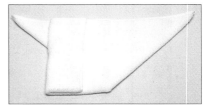

5 Then fold in another third. You will now have a thick central panel to go between your baby's legs, with two triangular 'wings' to fasten neatly round her tummy with a couple of safety pins.

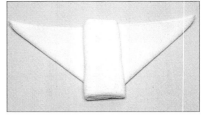

For a larger baby, you can use the 'kite' fold.

1 Lay the nappy on a flat surface so that it forms a diamond shape.

2 Bring each of the left and right hand points in to the centre of the nappy so that the two edges are touching (this forms the 'kite').

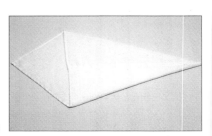

NAPPY RASH

NAPPY RASH CAN BE CAUSED BY	TO HELP AVOID OR TREAT IT
Substances in the urine reacting with bacteria in the faeces to irritate the skin	Change your baby's nappy frequently – even more often than usual if you see any signs of redness on her skin. If a rash has developed, applying a nappy rash cream can help it to heal.
The baby's skin being damp	Dry her bottom thoroughly when you change her. Leave her to kick without a nappy on at as many changes as you can. Using a barrier cream can help stop dampness. So can leaving off plastic pants.
Using soap or baby wipes	Use warm water and cotton wool instead.
Using strong detergents or fabric conditioner to wash cloth nappies	Use mild (non-biological) detergents and don't bother with fabric conditioner. Make sure the nappies are rinsed thoroughly.
Thrush	A nappy rash that remains red and sore, despite frequent nappy changes and plenty of fresh air, may be caused by thrush. See your doctor or health visitor.

'The first time Emma had nappy rash I thought I was a terrible mother. When I found out how common it was I felt better. Leaving her nappy off helped her bottom to heal.'

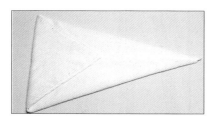

3 Fold the top point down to the centre, so that you have a straight edge along the top.

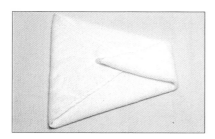

4 Fold the bottom point up towards the centre. How far you fold it will depend on your baby's size.

Most parents who use terry nappies use one-way nappy liners which allow wetness to pass through them into the nappy, but not back onto their baby's skin. You can either use disposable liners or washable fabric liners. Liners also prevent the nappy from becoming heavily soiled.

WHAT'S IN A NAPPY?

IN THE FIRST 2–3 DAYS, BABY POO IS:
black, tarry and sticky (meconium)

FROM 3–5 DAYS
greenish-brown and semi-fluid ('changing stools')

IN A BREASTFED BABY FROM ABOUT DAY 5
it's bright yellow, very loose, smelling like slightly sour milk

IN A BOTTLE-FED BABY FROM ABOUT DAY 5
it's light brown, formed and smelling more like ordinary stools

Both breastfed and bottle-fed babies may occasionally have greenish stools. This is nothing to worry about, but if it happens over several days, it may be worth checking with your doctor.

If you notice blood in the nappy, see your doctor.

LOOKING AFTER YOURSELF

There is no doubt that caring for a new baby is hard work – you may find yourself more tired than you've ever been before. Find ways of being pampered, so that you'll stay strong.

Your new baby will be depending on you to meet all her needs: warmth, comfort, food, security. The distinction between day and night is not a factor for her, but going without sleep is tough on you!

During the first week or two after birth, you may also find your emotions fluctuating enormously. Chance comments can be deeply upsetting, total euphoria and boundless energy can give way to tearful lack of confidence in yourself. This is caused by the huge hormonal changes that your body is undergoing.

Although it may seem to go on forever, this phase does soon pass. It can be very reassuring to know that most mothers experience this.

'If you don't look after yourself, everything hurts more.'

'The third and the seventh days were the worst: the slightest thing would upset me.'

Keep on top of things by trying these ideas:
• Accept all offers of help. Sometimes just having someone in to keep an eye on the baby while you soak in the bath can work wonders. Having support does not mean you aren't being a good mother. Your physical recovery will be quicker if you don't overload yourself.

'My sister offered help but I was afraid she would think I was lazy. Then I got an infection. Next time? I'll accept all the help I'm offered.'
• Rest when your baby rests. For once, let the housework go. Someone else can always catch up with it. Encourage helpers to do the housework while you spend time with the baby.
• Arrange for someone that you get on with to come and stay. You could arrange for a relative to help after the first week or so, giving you time to adjust to the baby on your own first.
• Stock up plenty of nutritious foods to keep your energy levels stable. Things like pasta, wholemeal bread, baked beans, cheese and fruit will give you long-lasting energy. Try to eat regularly, keeping plenty of simple snacks to hand so you can grab something to eat while you feed the baby.
• Drink lots of fluids, but go easy on the caffeine.

IN AN HOUR YOUR SUPPORTER COULD:
• hold the baby while you bath/shower
• let you get to the shops alone
• give you an hour's snooze
• let you go for a walk with your partner
• take your baby to the park in the pram
• make sandwiches for you and wash up
• let you choose a new cot without interruptions
• give you time to ring your friends.

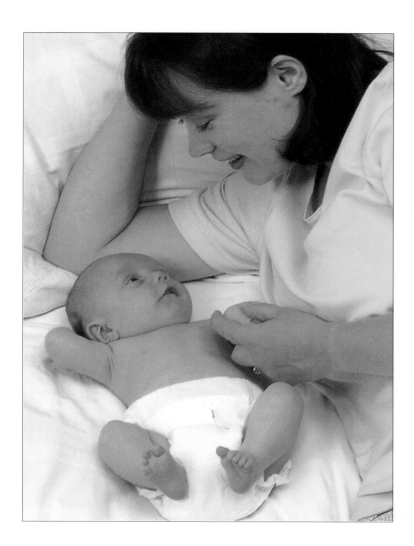

PARTNER'S CHECKLIST:

- be at home with the new baby as much as possible
- act as a go-between for your partner
- give plenty of emotional support, and don't question mood swings
- do the housework
- find out what she wants
- try to understand the huge changes in her life
- pamper her.

BE PREPARED FOR:

- mood swings
- tiredness times ten
- wanting to drink gallons of fluids while breastfeeding
- feeling that all you are doing is feeding
- everyone being an expert on your baby and all saying something different.

VISITORS

'I found friends dropping in far more difficult than I acknowledged.'

One of the pleasures of having a new baby is showing her off, but make sure your eagerness to see people doesn't work against you.

Ask friends to phone first rather than just dropping in, so you don't get snowed under with visitors. If you're tired, put the answering machine on, or pop a note on the door to the effect of: 'Mum and baby resting, please ring later. Thanks!'

You may prefer, in these very early days, to breastfeed alone. Often women like to take shirt and bra off to feed until they are proficient. If your baby needs to feed when there are visitors, perhaps your partner could steer them into the kitchen for a cup of tea so that you can breastfeed in private.

Hopefully your partner (if you have one – or what about asking your mother or a sister to stay with you?) will be able to spend time with you, getting to know your baby.

You definitely need a lot of help in these early weeks, so make sure you get it.

A BABY WITH PROBLEMS

When parents are first given the news that their baby isn't completely healthy or able, they may experience a mixture of feelings, either one after the other, or all at once.

Almost all parents at some time find it hard to cope with their babies, and almost all babies experience problems of some kind. Some parents, though, find themselves having to cope with a different degree of problems because their baby is suffering from an illness or a disability or a learning disorder that is going to affect him into the future.

HOW YOU MIGHT FEEL

Peter describes how he and Anna reacted to the news: 'At first we were shocked and numb, we just couldn't take it in. In fact, we didn't really believe it. We kept asking the doctors if they were sure. When we finally realised that there wasn't any doubt, we felt this overpowering grief and sadness. I suppose in a way we were mourning the loss of the baby we were expecting and hoping for. We felt angry too. It seemed so unfair. Why our baby? Why us?'

Feelings of confusion, anger and bitterness are common among parents whose baby has been born with a disability or other problem. It's also not unusual to find it difficult to relate to the baby at first, although for most parents this ultimately gives way to feelings of extra fierce love and protectiveness. Parents also often feel guilty about their baby's condition, asking themselves what they might have done to cause it, even when they have been told that they're not in any way to blame.

If your baby has been born with a disability, it will take time for you to come to terms with what's happened. Although at first you may feel that you'll never be able to adjust, eventually you will almost certainly come to accept the situation, and be able to see past the problem to your baby, who needs all the love and care that every baby needs, although possibly in a different form. But this won't happen overnight, and you may experience setbacks along the way. Don't rush yourself – take all the time you need.

TIME TO TALK

Many parents whose baby has a disability find that they need two things above all – information about the problem to help them understand it, and someone to talk to to help them cope with their feelings. Some find that it helps to have more than one source of information and more than one listening ear. Talking to medical professionals, a religious adviser, each other, can all help in different ways. In particular, it can be especially helpful to talk to other parents of children who have the same condition. These parents know better than anyone what it's like and are often more than willing to share their experiences and to support others who are coping with the same situation. For many conditions there are support groups whose members are happy to give others the benefit of their experiences. Your hospital doctor or GP should be able to give you details of these groups if you need them (or see the useful addresses at the back of this book).

One sort of talking that can be especially difficult is telling family and friends about what has happened. Anisha found that the best way of dealing with this was to tell everyone as soon as possible. 'It actually helped to tell people because it made it real. And having to explain what was wrong to them helped me to understand it more clearly too.'

COMING TO TERMS AND COPING

Although it can take a while, most parents whose baby has a disability do in time come to accept the situation and develop ways of coping with it. Many have found these strategies helpful:
• Take things one day at a time.
• Tackle problems individually, rather than trying to deal with them all at once.
• Redefine achievements, and let yourself be encouraged by small signs of progress even if they're agonisingly slow to happen.
• Make plans for dealing with setbacks, such as expected progress not being made.
• Take regular breaks from looking after your baby and do something special for yourself.

PREMATURE BABIES

If a baby is born before 37 weeks, he is classified as premature. His condition and the type of care he needs will depend on how soon before 37 weeks he's born.

Premature babies may look very thin and bony. Their skin is often thin too, and may be a dark red colour. They may be covered in dark downy hair. If they're very premature, they won't have any of this hair, nor any eyebrows and eyelashes. Those born before 26 weeks may not be able to open their eyes.

Premature babies need to be cared for in a special care baby unit. Because they lack fat, they need to be helped with keeping warm. They also often have to be helped with breathing because their lungs aren't sufficiently mature. They probably won't have developed the sucking reflex, so may need to be fed through a tube, although some of them can lap milk from a tiny cup. They're also vulnerable to infection.

If your baby needs to be in special care, being as involved as possible in looking after him, and talking to and stroking him, can help make you feel better about it.

If your baby has to stay in hospital for several weeks, it can be difficult to cope with the demands of spending time at the hospital and the demands of other parts of your life. One way of dealing with this conflict is to let things go that can be let go for a while or find someone to help with them. It can also help if you can share the hospital visiting with your partner, rather than having one of you spending all the time at the hospital and the other being at home or at work.

YOUR BABY FROM 1–3 MONTHS

By four weeks, you'll probably find there's a kind of rhythm in your relationship with your baby that sets the beat of things to come. Babies tune in to what you do, and of course, you tune in to your baby too.

By the time you and your baby have known each other for a month you'll have become familiar with each other's little ways. Lisa's baby now seems to know when a feed is coming: 'He starts to thrash his arms around and look excited now when I lift up my T-shirt!'. Some of your life together will be predictable – you know he wakes three or four times a night, and he knows that when he does, you will take him to you and let him feed.

Whether you are calm or anxious, slow or quick, quiet or chatty your baby will come to expect this of you. Babies in turn also seem to be calm or anxious, slow or quick, quiet or chatty – and any number of other characteristics – and by now you'll be starting to know how your personalities 'fit'.

Already, if you do something your baby doesn't expect, he will become worried or cry. In experiments, babies whose normally smiley mothers responded blankly to them, got very upset and cried. Their expectations had been shattered and they were hurt and confused.

COMMUNICATION

From the first few weeks babies have wordless conversations. As you talk, your baby's body stills and he listens, yet in the silence that follows, his whole body becomes more active. He's answering you, joining in. The two of you are communicating. His vocal chords are not developed sufficiently to make any sounds, beyond the odd gurgle, but just a few short weeks are enough to initiate him into the basic building block of good conversation – which is taking turns.

Something of a watershed occurs between four and six weeks. Your baby, whom you have been treating as though he were social, finally becomes social. He begins to respond to you as a person. He begins to smile. Many babies smile

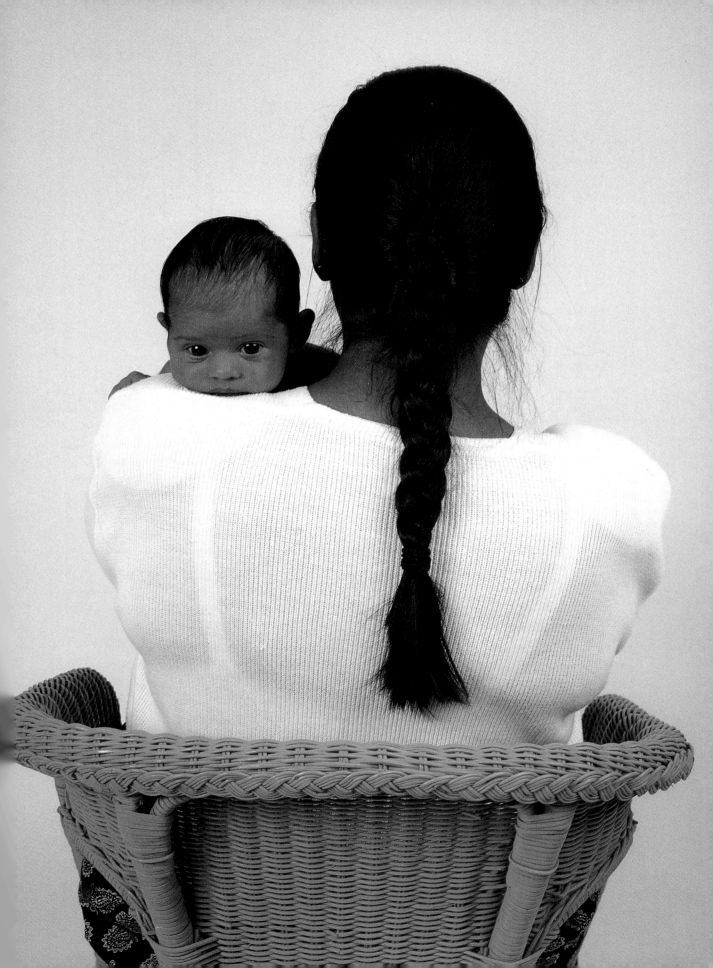

before four weeks and many mothers are not prepared to believe it's 'just wind'. But your pre-four week old smiling baby is unlikely to be smiling at you – it's a real smile all right, in the sense that the mouth is turned up at the corners, but it's not a smile of recognition, it's not a social smile. However, it soon will be if you keep treating it like one. Once your baby cottons on to the notion that smiling gets him your attention he'll do it more and more.

For the first month of life babies can only use one of their senses at a time. Suddenly, round about four to six weeks, your baby discovers that things that he sees may make noises and things which he can hear can also be looked at. He will start to turn towards sound. A few weeks later he will begin to make cooing sounds in response to social play – he's put together the idea of smiling and chatting – the visual and the verbal elements of good conversation.

New discoveries

Now he has made the connection between seeing and talking it will be a number of years before he will learn how not to see and talk at the same time. For now he will have to talk about everything as it happens, and if you can't listen then he'll talk to himself. The way you respond to him lets him know whether talking is worthwhile.

Another great discovery that your baby makes at this time are his hands. But at first he has no idea that they belong to him. They are just one more toy. As he thrashes his arms, exercising the muscles, one hand will find the other and your baby will pull, prod, squeeze and unfold his fingers, just as he would with any other toy. Perhaps the most surprising thing is that your baby will not even think to look at them as he plays. But when you have only just learnt to co-ordinate looking and listening, co-ordinating looking and playing is still a way off.

But soon he'll catch sight of his hands at play and after only another four to six weeks your baby will make the connection – he is the one who is pulling this fascinating toy about and the toy is him. He is ready to co-ordinate looking with doing. Now he will deliberately bring his hands up so that he can see them when he is lying on his back, or in his bouncer and make them do all manner of absorbing gymnastics. Hands make a brilliant first toy because even when they are dropped they have a habit of remaining nearby ready for another play.

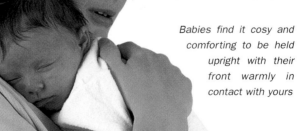

Babies find it cosy and comforting to be held upright with their front warmly in contact with yours

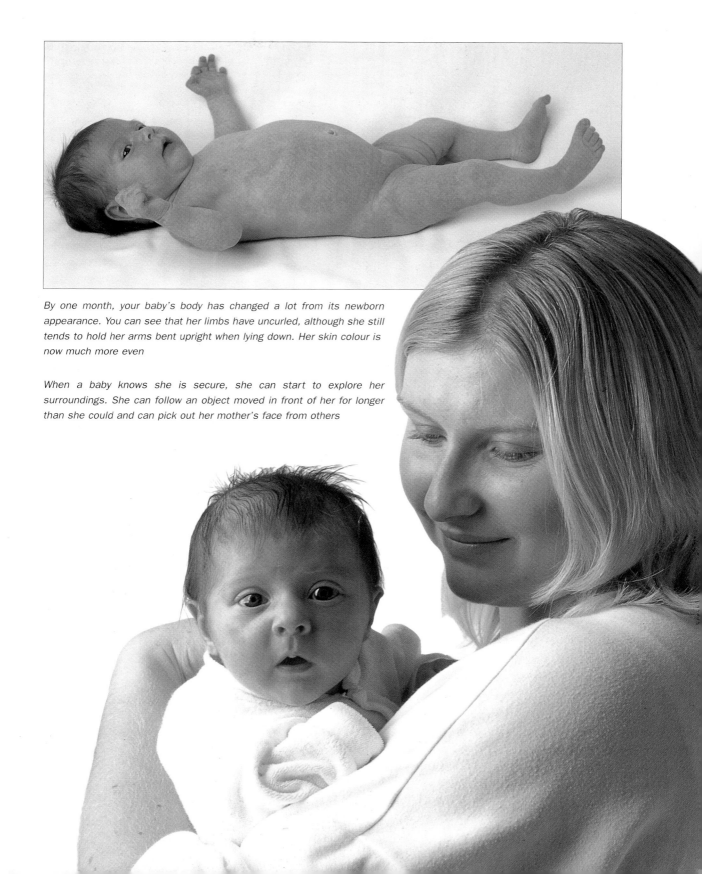

By one month, your baby's body has changed a lot from its newborn appearance. You can see that her limbs have uncurled, although she still tends to hold her arms bent upright when lying down. Her skin colour is now much more even

When a baby knows she is secure, she can start to explore her surroundings. She can follow an object moved in front of her for longer than she could and can pick out her mother's face from others

DIARY OF A ONE-MONTH-OLD

Daisy is six weeks old. Her parents are Sophie and Will. Sophie has given up work to look after Daisy. Will is out at work during the day.

Most of Sophie's time is taken up with looking after Daisy. 'She's the priority,' she says. 'I don't have much time for other things. I go to put the washing on, then Daisy needs something, then three hours later I realise that I still haven't put the washing on.' Sophie tries not to let this bother her. 'It's irritating, but I just say, oh well, never mind.'

5am

Daisy wakes for a feed, and goes back to sleep again straight away.

8am

Sophie gets up, has her shower, gets dressed and has breakfast. Will will have left for work any time in the last couple of hours.

8.30am

Daisy wakes up and Sophie gets her dressed.

9am

Daisy has another feed. She usually feeds about four or five hourly during the day. Sophie changes her nappy and Daisy goes back to sleep. Sophie, who is bottle-feeding Daisy, makes up a 24-hour supply of bottles in one batch.

10am

Daisy sleeps for most of the morning. Sophie either uses this time to do jobs around the house or she takes Daisy out shopping or to visit friends. 'Seeing people is important, and I try and do it most days – I need to have some adult contact,' she says. 'I find it quite easy to take Daisy out now, though it took me a bit of time at first to remember what to take with me, and I kept having to go back for things. But you learn, and it all comes together.' Nonetheless, Sophie finds that she can't do things spontaneously. As she puts it, 'I can't just pop somewhere, like out for a drink' – something her friends without children don't always appreciate.

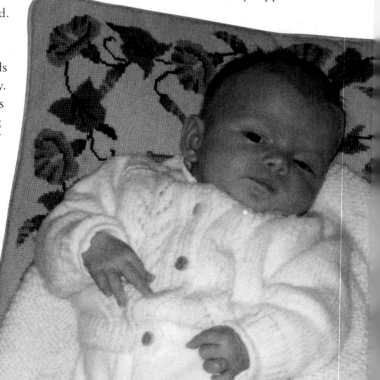

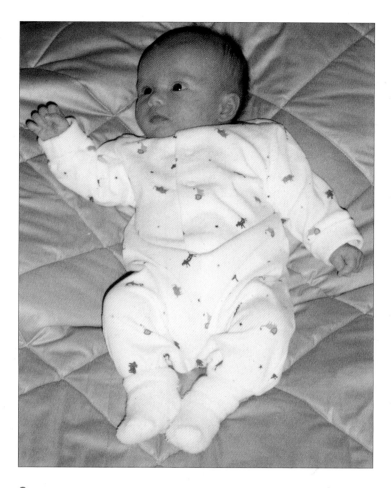

5.30–6pm

Bathtime. 'At first it took me two hours to bath her, but now I can do it quite quickly,' says Sophie. She has found that her confidence in looking after Daisy has grown tremendously. Although she was worried about the thought of caring for a baby before Daisy was born, she now feels that she instinctively knows what's right for Daisy, and feels confident in her intuition that she is doing the right thing.

6pm

Will comes home sometime between six and eight and Sophie is glad to hand Daisy over to him. Daisy tends to be unsettled and fretful in the evening and wants feeding every hour or two. Will holds her and feeds her and talks to her, while Sophie cooks supper for them both.

2pm

Daisy has another feed. She tends to stay awake for most of the afternoon, and prefers sitting in her bouncy chair to lying in her pram. She likes to look at things and she follows Sophie with her eyes. Sophie thinks that Daisy can now recognise her by sight rather than by smell or sound. Best of all, Daisy likes to be held, so Sophie holds her, talks to her and plays with her. In the few weeks since she was born, Daisy has become more alert, more robust and more aware of her body. She can support her head quite well and she can do more with her hands, reaching for and trying to grab things. And she has a definite personality. 'She's very strong-willed,' Sophie says.

9pm

Sophie puts Daisy in her crib. 'You can tell when she's really tired because she goes like a rag doll,' she says. She used to let Daisy go to sleep in her pram then transferred her to her crib when she went to bed herself, but she's now trying to get Daisy to recognise the bedroom as the place to sleep at night. Daisy usually goes to sleep at around 10pm and doesn't wake till four or five in the morning.

Sophie has found looking after Daisy easier than she expected. 'You just get used to it,' she says. 'You learn without realising.' She can't now imagine not having Daisy. 'All I want to do is be with her. I enjoy everything about it.'

STEP BY STEP DRESSING

Dressing a baby has been likened to trying to put an octopus into a string bag so that none of the legs stick out. The difference is that the octopus won't scream at you while you do it.

In the first month or two, babies often hate being undressed and howl in protest when you take their clothes off. By the time they're two or three months old, though, they've usually discovered that it's quite nice being unclothed, and enjoy being left to kick without any clothes or a nappy on.

When you change your baby's clothes, make sure that the room is warm, and that you have everything you need to hand before you start. It can be quite panic-inducing, when your baby is screaming about being undressed, to realise that you've forgotten her clean vest. If you smile at your baby and talk or sing to her as you dress her, it may make both of you feel more relaxed. Some nuzzles and kisses can help too.

GETTING DRESSED

It'll be some time before your baby is able to co-operate in moving her limbs in the direction you need them to go in order to dress her. For the moment, therefore, you'll have to move her limbs gently for her.

1 Lay your baby in a clean nappy on a changing mat. Bunch up her vest around the neck opening, and stretch the opening wide, so that you have a circle of fabric (vests with envelope necks will open widest). Position the back edge of the opening at the top of her head. Keeping the fabric well off her face, slip the front edge quickly over her face and under her chin. Lift her head slightly and slide the back of the

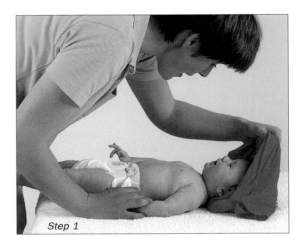

Step 1

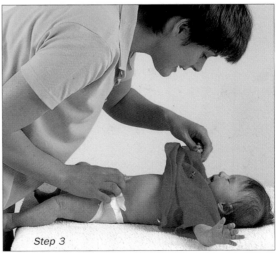

Step 3

vest down to the back of her neck. Alternatively, you can position the front edge of the opening under her chin and take the vest backwards over her head. Small babies often hate having clothes pulled over their heads, so this can be the worst part of dressing them. If it becomes a real problem, you can try using a wrap-over vest instead.

2 Still with the vest bunched up round her neck, stretch one armhole open with the fingers of one hand. With the other hand hold your baby's arm and guide her hand through the armhole so that you can take her hand with your fingers. Keeping hold of her hand, ease the vest up to her shoulder with your other hand. Do the same with the other armhole.

3 Pull the vest down. If it has poppers, hold your baby's feet in one hand to lift her bottom up slightly, and pull the back of the vest under her bottom. Do up the poppers.

PUTTING ON A STRETCH SUIT

1 Lay her stretch suit out flat on its back with its poppers undone, and put your baby on top of it.

2 Gather up one sleeve of the stretch suit and stretch the cuff open with the fingers of one hand. With the other hand, hold your baby's arm and guide her hand through the cuff so that you can take hold of her hand with your fingers. With your free hand, pull the sleeve up over her arm. Do the same with the other arm.

3 One at a time, bunch up the legs of the stretch suit and put the toes of the suit over your baby's feet, then pull the legs of the suit up over her legs. If the suit doesn't have feet, stretch the leg cuffs open and lift them over your baby's feet. (Some parents do it the other way round, legs first, then the sleeves.)

4 Do up the poppers – if you start from the bottom you may be less likely to miss one out and have to start again.

Now you're all done – pick your baby up and give her a big cuddle!

WASHING CLOTHES

Babies can generate an unbelievable amount of washing, and you can find yourself spending a lot of time keeping your baby's clothes clean.

- Some babies suffer skin reactions to washing products, including fabric softeners. If you suspect that your baby does, try using a mild, non-biological product.
- Be careful not to use too much detergent, or the clothes might be left stiff and itchy.
- Make sure you rinse the clothes thoroughly so that no traces of detergent are left in them.
- Dry the clothes outside if you can to help keep them soft. If you can't, giving them ten minutes in the tumble drier if you have one will keep them softer than just air drying them indoors. Drying them on a radiator will leave them particularly stiff.
- To help prevent stains becoming fixed, soak dirty clothes before you wash them. Sometimes soaking in cold water can be enough, or make up a cold detergent solution (keep any buckets or bowls away from toddlers). You may find that you're adding your own clothes to the bucket too.

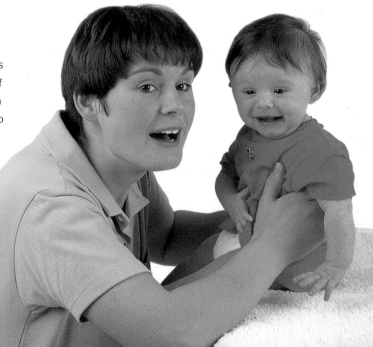

FEELINGS AND PHYSICAL SKILLS

Head, arms and legs all come together gradually, as your baby learns to move muscles in the way he wants.

Babies learn to control their bodies from the head downwards and from the middle outwards. By the time your baby is one month old he will have learnt how to support his incredibly heavy head for a short time – at least so long as you keep him upright and don't move. At the same time he's working towards control of his arms. Whenever you put him down awake he will thrash his limbs around – more his arms than his legs.

He's busy exercising his still feeble muscles, ready for the time when he can reach out for what he wants.

Between four and six weeks your baby will smile at you for the first time. It's a sign that he has noticed the difference between people and things. Finally there seems to be someone there! A few weeks after you celebrate his first smile he'll begin to coo socially. Before this you may have made all the running, but now he's ready for his first chat. He's learning to take it in turns. He coos, you listen; you talk, he listens.

'Before the first real smile, Minnie's eyes rolled up and you knew it was just wind. But now her eyes are really focused on me when she smiles and it's just a joy!'

FACING UP TO YOUR BABY

When you talk to or feed your baby he will gaze at you, gradually looking more alert. He's focusing on your face because it's curvy, it moves and has areas of high contrast, and babies love all those things. It's also about 20cm away, the distance at which he can focus best, which helps. But no matter what the reason, focusing on faces is a smart move because faces tell him much more about what's going on than, say, a kneecap. Your face is his gateway into the social world. From your face he will learn about smiling, talking and emotions.

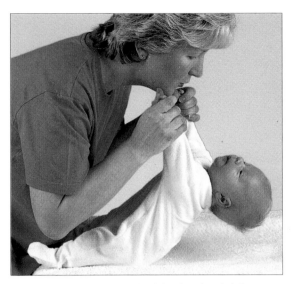

At eight weeks, Grace can hold her head up briefly...

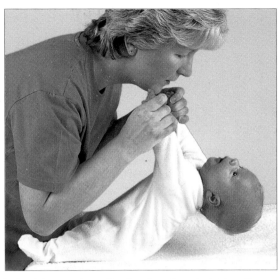

but not for very long. Head and neck control takes time

It is also a mirror of his importance. It's very hard to hide your true feelings from your baby. If you can't love him straight away, and many parents can't, don't try to hide behind a big smile – your baby will see through it, and the mixed message of looking happy and feeling sad will confuse him. Better to be honest with him and yourself. If your lack of loving is a problem for you talk it through with a good listener or talk to your baby about it – he can't understand a word you say, but his response to you may bring you closer to love.

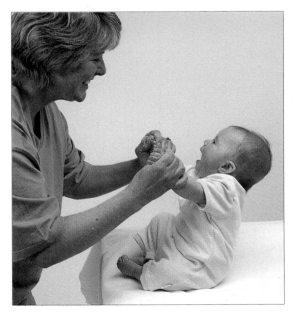

Rosie, who's two months older...

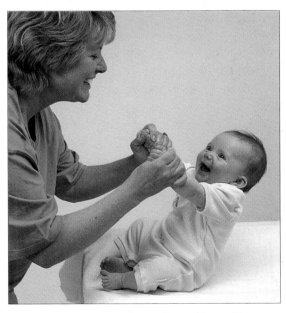

has developed strong neck muscles and loves this game

ESTABLISHED FEEDING

In the first few weeks of your baby's life, new feeding skills have to be learnt, both by you and the baby. Getting good at it can take time but it will come.

Preparing bottle-feeds is time-consuming until you know what you're doing, and with breastfeeding, you may have needed a few attempts to get the positioning right before settling down to a feed. The first weeks may have been chaotic and disorganised — probably stressful at times — and they will definitely have been unpredictable.

By the time six or eight weeks have passed, though, you should start to see a difference. Although life with a baby may still be unpredictable, you should be able to see some progress. The changes may be gradual but you should be noticing:

'It was only when I felt I had become competent that I was comfortable about feeding in public.'

'I wanted to breastfeed and I'm glad I persevered, as it's so simple now.'

• **A growing confidence in your ability to feed your baby**

Perhaps there were days when you worried that he wasn't getting enough milk, or considered visiting the doctor when he seemed to bring back the whole of his feed. By now these issues can be put into a context, as you are getting to know your baby.

• **A developing familiarity with your baby's cries**

You can probably tell the difference now between crying for a feed, and crying when he's bored and wants a different view, or a cuddle.

It's likely that you felt slightly bewildered at the beginning. Is it hunger? But he was only fed an hour ago. Is it boredom? Is it wind? As your experience grows, your ear will be getting more tuned in to your baby's needs.

• **A noticeable weight gain**

His weight gain may be erratic, but you should be able to see it moving up the scale,

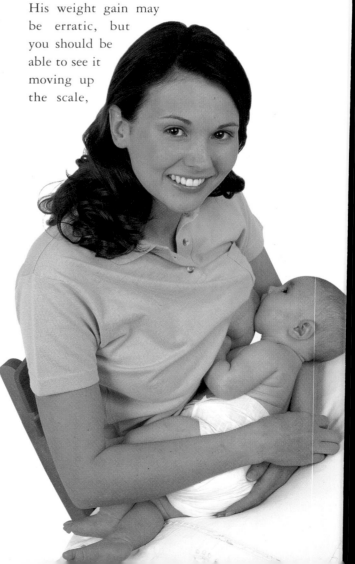

confirming that you are doing things right. Babies do not all gain weight at the same speed, so concentrate on an overview of the weight gain, rather than worrying if one week's gain is slightly less than the previous one.

• **An awareness of your baby's demanding times**

Some babies want to feed and feed at certain times of the day. Once you become familiar with this pattern, you can plan around it.

If you are breastfeeding, for example, you may find that your baby feeds a lot during the evenings. This happens because the milk producing hormone (prolactin), works at its best when you are resting, so by the evening, particularly if you have been busy all day, it takes longer to make milk. Try resting for a couple of hours during the afternoon.

TROUBLE-FREE BREASTFEEDING

You'll probably find that by now you are able to feed in a much more relaxed way. You should not be experiencing any discomfort, and the feeds will probably be shorter, as your baby grows and becomes more efficient at breastfeeding. Whilst you may have experienced some uncomfortable bouts of engorgement (swollen breasts) while your milk supply was getting established, these troubles should have passed by now.

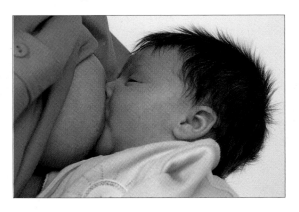

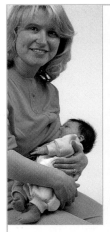

YOU KNOW YOU ARE GETTING THERE WHEN:

- you still listen to all the conflicting advice but start to trust your own judgement
- you don't fret when someone says to your crying baby: 'Is your mummy starving you then?' You just raise your eyebrows
- you can latch the baby on without thinking about it
- you know you can breastfeed discreetly when out and about
- you stay calm when your baby is crying for a feed, and you have to wait for the bottle to warm up.

BY NOW YOU WILL HAVE DECIDED WHICH FEEDING METHODS SUIT YOU BOTH

Leave guilt behind now and enjoy your baby, if all is going well. Things can turn out differently from what you expected. Some mothers don't like the idea of breastfeeding, but take to it immediately. Others have problems getting started, and decide to give up. Some mothers make an informed decision to bottle-feed their baby because it is the method which suits them best. Whatever choice you make, don't feel guilty about it.

However, if you feel that you didn't want to take the path that you are now travelling along, then you may benefit from talking to a breastfeeding counsellor. She's not only there to get breastfeeding established, but would be happy to talk to you if your breastfeeding experience was not a happy one, or if you now want to stop breastfeeding.

BABY MASSAGE

There's nothing quite like massage for soothing and calming both you and your baby. It can be done from about two months, ideally after bathtime in preparation for sleep.

Massage is a wonderful way of bonding with your baby and particularly good if this is a second or third baby who doesn't get a lot of special time alone with you, apart from feeding. Remember, you don't have to do a full massage every time – if you're in a hurry, just do the favourite bits. It will help you to unwind and you'll both look forward to it as a restful, reassuring moment of calm in your busy day.

BASIC TOUCH

The basic movement to use is a firm but gentle stroke with either the flat pads of your fingers or the whole palm of your hand. Small circular movements with the pads of your fingers can also be effective, as long as you don't tickle. Try not to break contact abruptly at any time. If you need to reach over and get a tissue, for example, keep the other hand on your baby's skin for reassurance. Try smoothing and squeezing your own arm to find out what feels nice – remembering that baby skin is more delicate and sensitive than yours. Too gentle a touch can be irritating and too hard will hurt.

BEGINNING

Have everything ready before you start. Find a warm, quiet place where you won't be interrupted and have everything to hand –

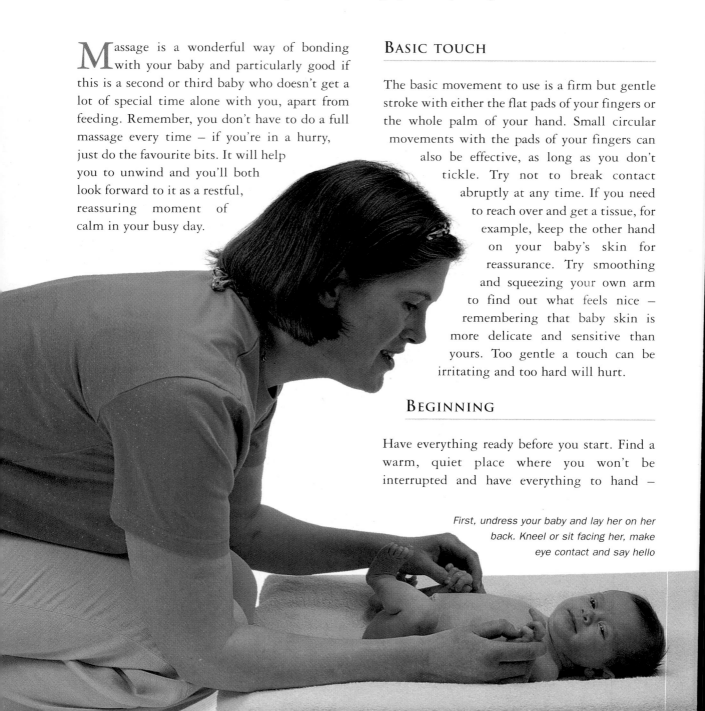

First, undress your baby and lay her on her back. Kneel or sit facing her, make eye contact and say hello

WHEN NOT TO MASSAGE

- Don't give a massage near feeding time (one hour before or after is best).
- Never wake a baby up for massage.
- Don't massage an ill or fractious baby.
- Wait 48 hours after immunisation jabs and then avoid the injection site.
- Don't massage over rashes or wounds without professional advice.
- Aromatherapy oils designed for adults should be avoided.
- Never use deep pressure when you massage a baby.

massage oil, tissues, a clean nappy and clean clothes. Baby massage is usually done on the floor, with the baby laid on a towel on top of a changing mat or folded blanket.

Remove any rings or bracelets, make sure fingernails are short and wash your hands in warm water, dry them, then rub together to make them nice and warm.

Undress your baby and lay her on her back, kneel or sit facing her and taking about half a teaspoon of oil (either a baby massage oil or any vegetable oil that smells nice) rub it over the palms of your warm hands. Use just enough oil to let your hands glide smoothly over the skin. Talk to your baby, make eye contact and tell her what you're going to do.

Stroke gently upwards, around the shoulders and smoothly back down. Repeat a few times, letting your baby's response guide you

SAY HELLO

First place your hands side by side, palm down, flat on the baby's tummy and stroke gently upwards, around the shoulders and smoothly back down to the toes. Then up again, over the body, round the shoulders and back to the toes. Repeat a few more times, making eye contact and talking gently, letting your baby's response guide you.

CHEST AND ARMS

Without applying more oil to your hands, place them together, palms down, side by side, on the baby's chest and gently press them down, round the chest and up again. From the same starting position, stroke up around the shoulders and down again, stroking the arms down towards the wrists. Repeat this movement two or three times, without getting any massage oil on the baby's hands (it will irritate her eyes if she rubs them).

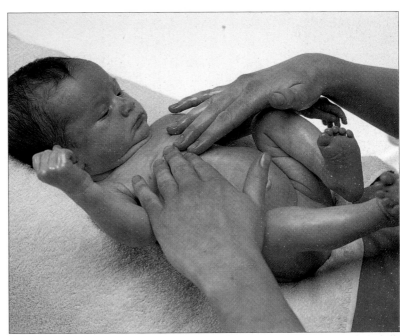

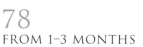
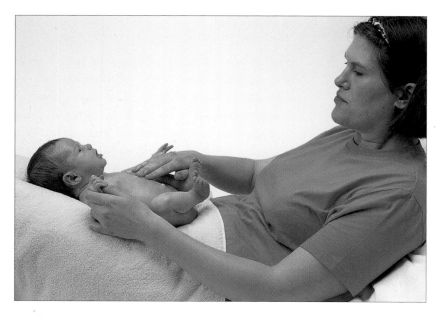

Rubbing small clockwise circles on the tummy can sometimes help a colicky baby. Clockwise movements are stimulating and anti-clockwise are calming

TUMMY

Put a little oil on your hands and make clockwise circles over the tummy with one hand and then, with the pads of two fingers, make small clockwise circles around the colon (beginning just up from the right groin, upwards to just under the ribs, across to the other side and down). Repeat a few times. This sometimes helps colicky babies. Then repeat the 'hello' strokes you began with, running your hands around the shoulders and back down to the toes. Turn your baby over.

LEGS

Apply a little more oil to your hands if needed and, starting with hands at either side of the base of

the spine, stroke up to the shoulders and back down to the toes a few times before smoothing each leg in turn.

Hold one of the baby's ankles in one hand and with the other hand, take hold of the top of the leg on the other side. Pull down gently but firmly and, as you get to the ankle, move your other hand up to the top of the leg on the same side, pulling down in the same way, while the first hand takes over holding the ankle. Repeat several times, swapping hands as you go. You may need to use a little more oil.

Go through the same massage on the other leg and then finish by running both hands up both legs at the same time, gliding right back down to the end of the toes in a satisfying way. Repeat this finishing stroke a few times.

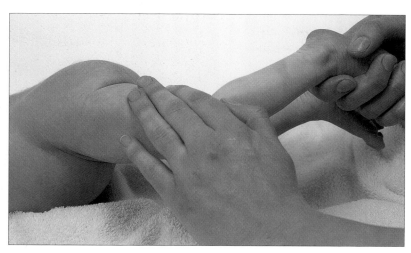

Hold one of the baby's ankles in one hand and with the other, smooth down the leg gently

FEET

With your thumb, rub small circles on the base of your baby's foot (anti-clockwise circles should calm her down). Massage her toes with small, circular movements too, pulling them gently. Repeat on the other foot and then 'finish off' with the same up and down the legs movement that you used before.

BACK

Put a little more oil on your hands and, starting with hands at either side of the base of the spine, stroke up to the shoulders and back down to the toes. Glide your hands back up the legs to either side of the base of the spine and repeat the movements on the back a few times. Using the pads of your thumbs, make little circles up both sides of the spine, smooth hands back down and repeat. Do not touch the actual spine itself, only massage at each side.

With the flat of the hand, make large anti-clockwise circles around the base of the back. Finish off with a few stroking movements – up the back, round the shoulders and back down to the toes.

Finally, wrap your baby in a clean, warm towel and give her a cuddle.

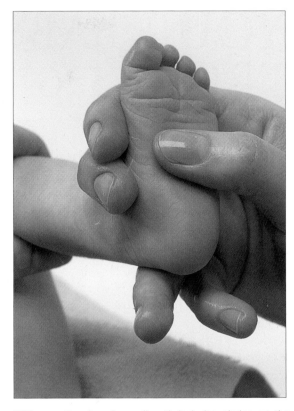

With your thumb, rub small anti-clockwise circles on the sole of your baby's foot. A firm touch won't tickle

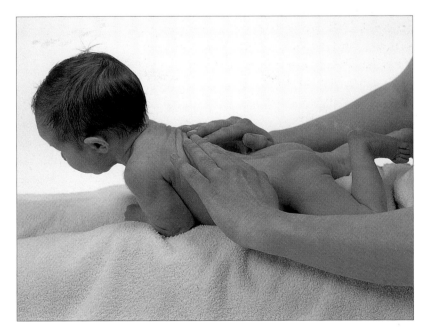

Starting with hands at either side of the base of the spine, stroke up to the shoulders and back down to the toes

YOUR BABY FROM 3–6 MONTHS

While the first 12 weeks of a baby's life are often known as 'the fourth trimester of pregnancy', a totally new phase seems to start after the third month.

Many mothers and fathers seem to emerge from the fog of new parenthood by about three months. For the first time since your baby was born, you may begin to see how you can co-ordinate caring for your baby with caring for yourself. And you may finally feel that you and your baby are acting as one, rather than against each other.

Co-ordination is very much the name of the game for your baby as well, because over the next few months they do learn to co-ordinate increasingly complex activities. Already your baby will have begun to co-ordinate her hands and her eyes, watching her hands as she squishes both palms together. But now, she's ready to start the long haul of co-ordinating her body with things outside by trying to swipe at objects in her view.

Her hands, which are normally kept closed, will begin to open up and she will begin to follow things out of sight by moving her head.

GRASPING

By three months your baby will be grasping for things – opening her hand, moving her arm in the right direction and closing her hand again – but she won't be able to catch hold of things. She needs you to hold them near her, give her time to reach out and then if she fails to grasp, put them into her hand.

Another ten weeks on and she's so familiar with her hands that she doesn't need to think about where they are. If she sees something she wants, she just has to keep her eyes focused on it and her hands can successfully reach out and close around it.

TRACKING

At the same time, babies can deliberately co-ordinate moving their heads and eyes to follow you as you move about the room. When you

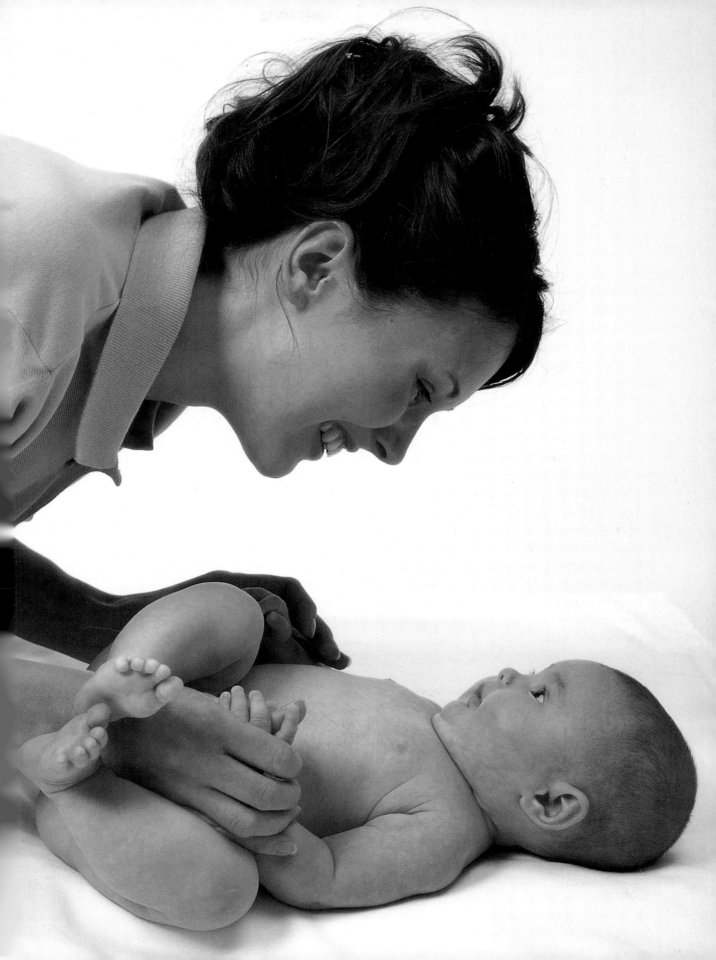

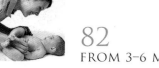

pull her up to sitting at three months your baby can bring her head with her and keep it balanced on her shoulders for a little while, even if you move her. So now you need only hold her shoulders when you bath and dress her.

Most three-month-olds can also lift their heads right up while lying prone. Later your baby will be able to lift her shoulders too. As she does these little press-ups, she will start to scratch at surfaces with her fingers – trying to pick up patterns from the carpet. At this stage, she doesn't yet know the difference between pictures and 3D objects.

BEGINNING TO TALK

At the same time as she's struggling to co-ordinate some things, your baby will begin the equally valuable task of differentiating between others. Up to now her chatting and smiling have kept each other company. But now she'll begin to chat more when you chat to her and smile more when you smile.

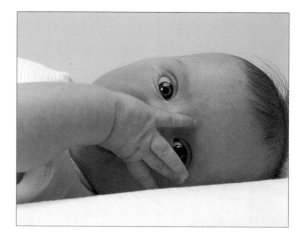

From three months your baby will begin to smile more broadly at people she knows, and by four months she will be restrained with other people and happy with you. She's beginning to discriminate between people as well.

At three to four months your baby coos delightedly when you talk to her, and also practises when alone, just for the sheer hell of it. She is excited by her growing ability to make a noise. At this age most of her sounds are open vowels: 'aaah' and 'oooh'. The first consonants – K, P, B and M – come a little later. By four to five months your baby will watch your face even if you aren't talking to her – she's so tuned in to sounds.

Your three month baby will be much more alert than before, and fascinated by human faces. Earlier she was just as likely to enjoy gazing at a picture of a face as at the real thing. Now she definitely prefers the living, breathing model.

She'll begin to enjoy the familiar routines of life – bathing, feeding and tickling – and will make welcoming movements as you prepare for these activities. Sudden loud noises will make your baby blink, screw up her eyes, turn away and start to cry. Predictability is comforting, but the unexpected is not.

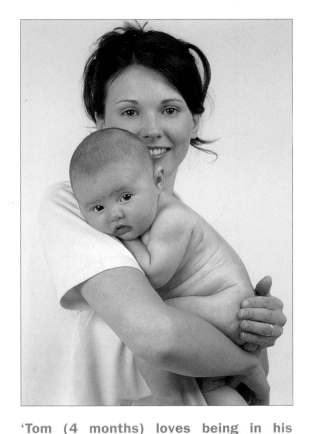

STIMULATING YOUR BABY

Babies of all ages enjoy experiences that stretch them a little, but not too much. At this age, when your baby is just beginning to use her hands to touch things or to grab and play with toys it's important to keep her interested. What she can use now is a wide variety of different toys and experiences, each a little different from the one before. So have two or three boxes containing different toys and swap them every few days. You could also let her examine safe household objects (a wooden spoon, plastic cups etc.) as well as toys – as long as you only let her have two or three objects to examine at once.

Vary the route that you walk, or the time that you go out, so that she sees different things along the way. And let her sit up in her special seat to watch you working.

'Tom (4 months) loves being in his pushchair, especially going places where there are animals, birds or children to watch and wave at.'

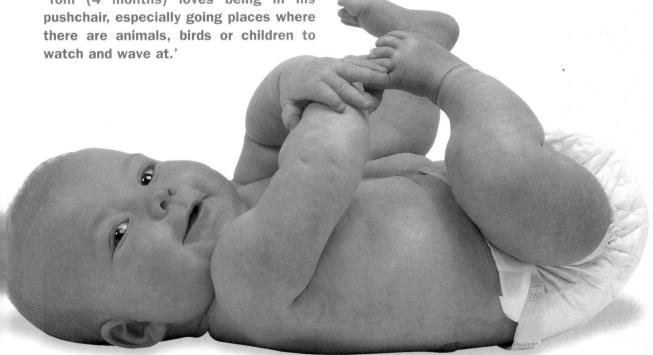

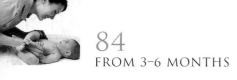
'Graham (4 months) spends half his waking time chewing his fingers as though fascinated by these clever "toys". He loves to play with them and watch what they do!'

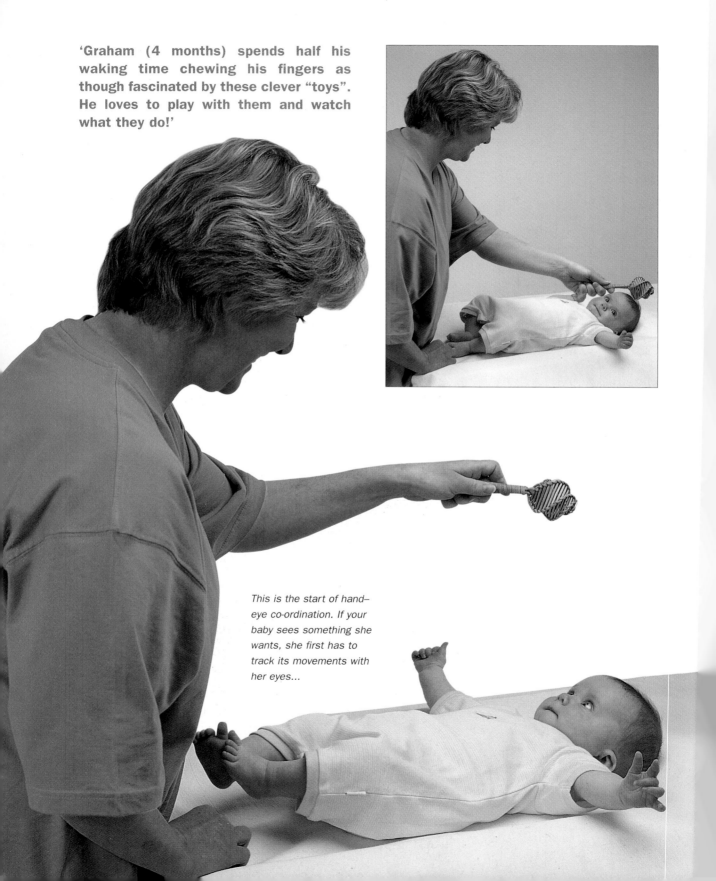

This is the start of hand–eye co-ordination. If your baby sees something she wants, she first has to track its movements with her eyes...

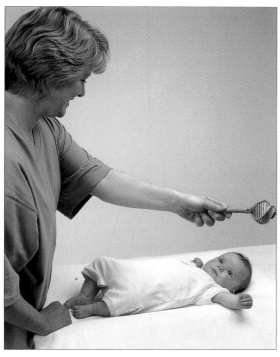

...and pretty soon, she will reach out a hand and curl her fingers around the desired object. This marks a big step forward in development

VISUAL PERCEPTION

Help her develop the beginnings of hand–eye co-ordination by holding a light toy or rattle about ten inches in front of her eyes and letting her focus on it. Then move the toy slowly and watch her 'track' it with her eyes, moving her head at the same time. Soon, she will reach out a hand to grasp the toy with her fingers.

It is now believed that 'shape constancy' is present at birth. We human beings are born with an in-built understanding that when we see an object from different angles or distances, we know that it hasn't actually changed shape, but that we're seeing it from a new perspective. At one time, child psychologists believed that a baby's brain was a complete blank at birth and that everything about the world needed to be learnt from scratch. Now, it seems that babies are born with a lot more abilities than was at first thought. It's not the babies that are getting cleverer, but the psychologists studying them!

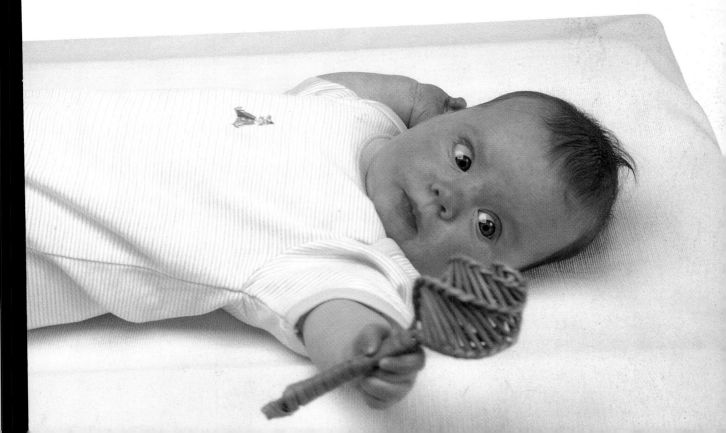

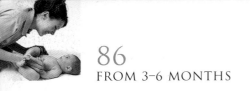

DIARY OF A THREE-MONTH-OLD

Madeleine is three months old. Her mother, Catherine, is still on maternity leave, but is returning to work in a month. Her father, Maher, is out at work during the day, but is going to take three months' leave to look after Madeleine when Catherine goes back to work. Madeleine will then go to a childminder.

Catherine is finding that Madeleine is changing by the week, and that she is having to adapt as her baby changes. She has adopted the philosophy of not trying to impose any routine on Madeleine or to alter her patterns at all, but is letting herself be led by Madeleine. 'I know other people do it differently, but this is the best way for us,' she says.

5–6am

Madeleine wakes and Catherine takes her into bed with her and Maher, and gives her a feed. They then all go back to sleep for a while.

6–7am

Madeleine wakes up again and is very lively and active. 'She laughs and smiles and is really happy,' says Catherine. 'It's very entertaining.'

7.30am

Catherine gets up and Madeleine plays lying on a mat under her baby gym while Catherine is getting herself dressed.

8am

Madeleine has another feed – she generally feeds every two or three hours during the day – then Catherine puts her in her bouncy chair while she tries to get on with domestic tasks. This doesn't always go down too well with Madeleine. 'I leave her in her bouncy chair when I need to do things around the house, but she doesn't like it, and she cries,' says Catherine. 'She likes to have my attention all the time.'

9–10am

Madeleine has a nap, often in her bouncy chair. She doesn't like to lie down in her cot during the day, and prefers to sleep in her chair, or car seat, or when she's being carried in her sling. Catherine is concerned that this isn't ideal, but feels that what matters most is that Madeleine has a sleep, wherever it is.

11am

Catherine and Madeleine go out. Catherine says that it's important to both her and Madeleine for them to get out every day, so they always go for a walk, or shopping, or to visit friends, including one friend Catherine made at her NCT antenatal class. Madeleine likes company and enjoys looking at faces and making eye contact. She has recently started very intently studying the faces of other babies she meets.

12.30–1pm

Catherine has her lunch and Madeleine has a feed.

2pm

Although she sleeps for a while during the afternoon, most of the time Madeleine is awake and wanting Catherine's attention. She's happy to look at her baby gym or her mobiles on her own for a little while, and is starting to reach towards them and to try and take hold of them, but she seems to get bored or frustrated after about quarter of an hour. So Catherine plays with her, walks around with her, talks to her or sings or plays music to her. Madeleine particularly enjoys music.

6–7pm

Catherine (or Maher if he's home) gives Madeleine a bath. Madeleine used to hate being

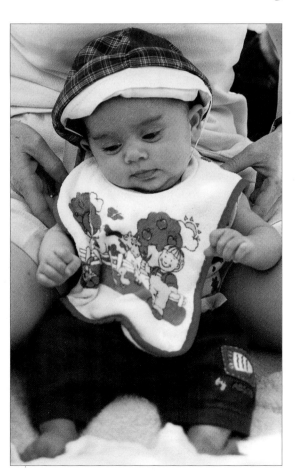

bathed, so Catherine kept baths to a minimum. Now she enjoys it, so she has a bath every day. She hasn't yet discovered the delights of a good kick and splash, though, preferring to lie still and watch Catherine. She also now enjoys being undressed and having her nappy changed.

7–8pm

Madeleine is often a bit cranky in the evening, and likes to be held or carried. Every other evening, Maher gives her a bottle of expressed breast milk, in preparation for when Catherine goes back to work. Catherine started expressing breast milk when Madeleine was about a month old.

8–9pm

Recently, Madeleine has started going to sleep earlier in the evening, and will now go to sleep as early as 8pm. Once she's asleep, she usually only wakes once for a feed (around midnight) during the night.

Catherine found the first couple of months with Madeleine exhausting and quite difficult, but things are easier now. Most of her time is taken up with looking after Madeleine and coping with the extra tasks that a baby generates – like washing. She delights in Madeleine's laughing and smiling and gurgling, and marvels at the way in which she's developing. But she admits to finding baby-centred activities 'a little boring at times', and misses things like reading and exercising, which she doesn't have time for at the moment. She also feels that in focusing on Madeleine, she has rather lost a sense of herself, which she's looking forward to regaining. But she has enjoyed discovering how being a parent has given her a new bond with other parents, and, best of all, she says, 'I love being a family'.

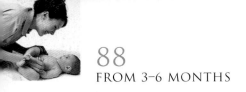

BECOMING PARENTS

Now that your life is filled with the responsibilities of being a parent, you'll wonder what on earth you did with all that time you had in your pre-baby days.

You may still be settling into the role of mother, still savouring using the words 'my son' or 'my daughter' and presenting your pride and joy to friends and family. It may seem very difficult to remember a time when your baby wasn't around.

You may also be surprised by the strength of feeling for your baby, although it may not have happened overnight. You may find that it takes time, but when that love is in place, it can sometimes be quite overwhelming. Before you gave birth, you may have been planning your return to work and looking forward to the challenge of being a working parent. Now you are exploring the possibilities of taking extended maternity leave, or even going part-time. You may also have been considering asking your parents to look after the baby for a night or so, while you get away with your partner. Now, you put it off, feeling secretly sure that you are the only one who can really look after her.

YOU AND YOUR PARTNER

'Having a baby has changed our relationship. We've had to cope together. The other person is the only one you really trust with your baby.'

Both you and your partner are probably enjoying the change in the family dynamic: a new baby to look after, a cementing of your relationship. With a new baby comes a new balance. As proud parents-to-be, you probably shared as much as possible of the pregnancy, going to antenatal classes together, reading up about pregnancy and birth, and being together when she was born.

The input from mother to baby is likely to be intense at this stage, particularly if you are breastfeeding. It is unlikely that you are back at work yet, so it's probable that you will be with the baby whilst your partner is out working during the day.

Being with a baby all day can be tiring and emotionally all-consuming and you may feel that you can't give as much to your partner because you are simply too tired. Often, new mothers are recovering from the physical impact of the birth and so are reluctant to make love, even if they did have the energy.

Your partner may be feeling the lack of sex as a kind of rejection, as well as feeling less adept

---

WAYS OF STAYING CLOSE:

- talk to your partner about your feelings
- listen to how your partner is feeling
- set aside some time together. Plan a weekly meal together with no TV, the answering machine on, and a takeaway to eat
- use touch (stroking, massage, holding hands) to reassure each other of affection, even if you aren't ready to make love
- leave your own expertise with the baby aside, and don't undermine him when he wants to be involved.

at caring for your baby than you are. Don't forget that it's his baby too. The more he looks after the newcomer, the more 'engrossed' he'll become – like you. Involved dads are far less likely to see the child as competition, although he may need your reassurance, in words, that he is still important to you.

And you may need him to be less of a lover and more of a protector: 'I'm less interested in sex now – it's not a priority any more, but it's lovely when it happens.'

POSTNATAL DEPRESSION

It is normal to feel tired, even exhausted at times, after the birth. You may feel tearful, irritable and anxious: in fact, it is believed that more than fifty per cent of women

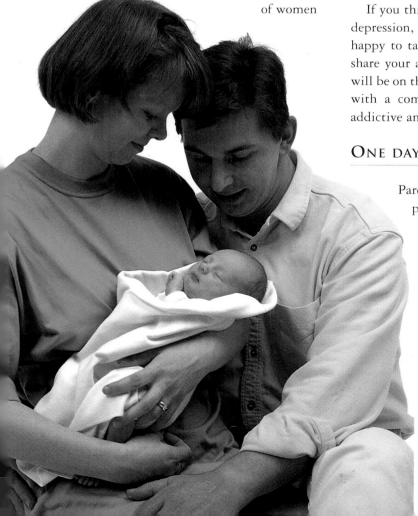

experience these symptoms, often known as the 'baby blues', in the first week after birth. Happily, these symptoms normally clear very quickly.

Postnatal depression (PND) is more severe than this. For most sufferers, the onset is within a month of giving birth though this may extend up to six months postpartum.

Some of the symptoms of PND are:
• Sadness
• Feeling a failure
• Finding it difficult to cope
• Finding it difficult to go out
• Anxiety
• Sleeplessness
• Loss of concentration
• Loss of appetite
• Extreme tiredness

If you think you are suffering from postnatal depression, your health visitor or GP will be happy to talk to you about it. The sooner you share your anxieties about this, the sooner you will be on the mend, and it will get better, often with a combination of counselling and non-addictive anti-depressants.

ONE DAY AT A TIME

Parenthood is often a combination of peaks and troughs, highs and lows. Responsibilities, tiredness, pressure from work can make it difficult at times, whilst the joys of seeing your baby smile, or seeing the growth of love between a new father and his baby, makes all the fatigue melt away.

Remember that this can be a stressful time and keep listening to your partner – try to be there for each other, enjoy the present and take each day as it comes.

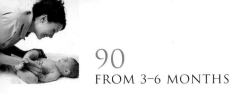

OUT AND ABOUT

Going out with a baby is a little different from popping into town on your own to pick up shopping. Once you were able to put on your jacket and swing into action, but going out as a twosome requires a little more preparation!

With a baby, outings take longer than you think to plan and organise. You'll have to pack the changing bag to meet all your baby's needs while you're out. Then the inevitable happens: the baby is sick on your shirt as you pick her up to put her in the sling. Or a dirty nappy is produced seconds before closing the front door. Be reassured that you are not the only one to despair of ever getting anywhere on time any more. Babies and deadlines don't sit at all comfortably together. If you are meeting someone, give an approximate time. Chances are, if she has a baby too, that she will appreciate the flexibility.

'Try to get out every single day'

A walk outside is going to make you feel better than staying at home and thinking that it wasn't worth the effort. Fresh air and exercise will give you a boost of energy, which is particularly useful during days and nights with little sleep. Your baby will benefit too: it's no old wives' tale that fresh air is good for you. The movement of the pram, or being in a sling, will probably send him to sleep quickly too, and give you some time for window shopping, or just gathering your thoughts in the park.

Getting to know other mothers, by going to a mother and baby group, or just by meeting casually, can result in lifelong friendships and give you the opportunity to talk to others who understand the ups and downs of your current life – because they're in the same boat.

AND IN THE EVENING, TOO

While your baby is still tiny and hasn't started solids, you have the ultimate mobile baby. You may feel that you don't want anyone else to look after him, but if you want to have a night out, why not take him along too?

There are plenty of non-smoking restaurants that welcome small babies, especially in the early evening when it's quiet. Some restaurants are particularly family friendly – perhaps your local Italian or Chinese restaurant is family run – your baby would probably be the star of the evening.

Making an effort to do something like this can make you feel part of the human race again, and should also give you time to talk to your partner. And the worst that can happen is that he won't settle and you'll have to leave early. Ask for a doggy bag and eat the rest at home!

TIPS

Make sure your changing bag is always ready to go – replace any used nappies, or stretch suits as soon as you come home. That way, you can be more spontaneous next time.

If you feel nervous about going out, particularly after a caesarean section, ask someone to come with you for the first couple of trips, until you feel more confident.

Many shops have lifts if they are multi-storey,

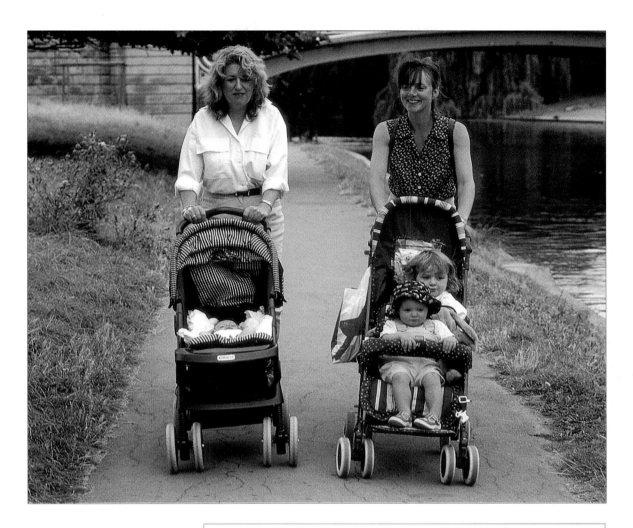

but they don't always advertise them. Always ask an assistant.

If your trip involves doors and shops that are hard to negotiate, take the baby in a sling.

Don't make shopping trips too lengthy. Decide to cut it short and go home before you start to get tired. Trips have a habit of dragging out longer than planned.

BREASTFEEDING OUT AND ABOUT

Now that you are breastfeeding proficiently, there is no reason why it should restrict your movements. With no special equipment needed, it's easy to breastfeed a baby away from home, although you may feel self-conscious at first.

Remember to wear breastfeeding-friendly clothes when out, such as baggy shirts and loose jumpers.

Cover your chest and your baby's head with muslin, or a scarf, or tuck him right inside your jumper.

Many stores have baby-feeding rooms if you prefer some privacy. Talk to other mums to find out where they are.

Remember, it's people who disapprove of breastfeeding in public that have the problem, not you.

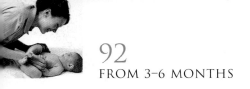

WORK AND BREASTFEEDING

How will you feed your baby if you have to go back to work before you've weaned him off the breast?

You may still be breastfeeding as your return to work draws closer. Is this a good time to wind it down? Some mothers like to 'have their bodies back' by the time they return to the workplace. Others plan to carry on breastfeeding by expressing their breast milk and arranging for someone else to give it to their baby in their absence. However, all the expressing, storing and freezing can seem very complicated.

There are various reasons why working mothers choose to carry on breastfeeding. Sometimes it's less complicated to continue, rather than switch feeding methods at this point. It also seems wise to keep as many aspects of a baby's life unchanged as possible, at a time when mother has to return to work. Anyway, if you and your baby both find a feed enjoyable and relaxing, it could become the ideal end to a busy working day. It's also worth continuing to give the best nutrition.

Alternatively, you can breastfeed when you are together, and arrange for your baby to be given formula milk while you are at work.

EXPRESSING

If you decide to express, you will need to build up a good supply of milk, which can be stored for use. As well as giving you time to build up a store, starting to express milk well in advance of your return to work means that your breasts will adjust to the change of pattern. You will also be good at expressing breast milk by the time you return. It would be wise to give yourself three to four weeks of preparation.

You also need to consider the practical aspects if you plan to express your milk at work. Your employer should help you find a private room while you need it. You'll need access to a fridge to store milk in during the day, and a cool box to transport milk from work to home.

CUTTING DOWN

If you are going to cut out breastfeeding in the middle of the day and replace it with formula feeds, you should leave three or four days between each feed that is dropped, so that your body can adapt gradually to the change. Depending on how many feeds you are dropping, you probably won't need a whole month, but you could use that time to get your baby used to feeding from a bottle or beaker.

STORING BREAST MILK

If you want to store breast milk, you can use:
• The refrigerator, for up to 24 hours
• The freezer compartment of the refrigerator, for up to seven days
• The freezer, for up to three months

Note that freezing breast milk does destroy some of the antibodies. It is not a good idea to freeze your milk for long periods as its properties are tailor-made specifically for your baby at each moment of its life. (Isn't nature wonderful?)

If you want to freeze a day's supply in the same container, you can add one batch to another in the fridge, but chill down the fresh milk first.

STORAGE CONTAINERS

Containers should be sterilised and dated. Try:
- Feeding bottles
- Covered ice-cube trays
- Sterile plastic bags (available from babywear departments and chemists)

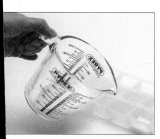

Storing milk in small quantities saves wastage and speeds up defrosting. You can freeze in ice-cube trays, if you like, then transfer the cubes into a sterile plastic bag.

Make sure that you leave space at the top of bottles, as the milk will expand when frozen.

TRANSPORTATION

If you are expressing away from home, make sure the milk is chilled at all times. You could use a cool bag with ice packs for travelling.

THAWING

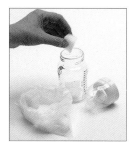

Breast milk should be thawed gradually, by holding the container under running water. It should not be thawed in the microwave, as this not only destroys some of the nutrients, but may also cause 'hot spots' which could burn your baby.

Defrosted milk can stay in the fridge for up to 24 hours, so long as it has not been warmed.

USEFUL TIPS:
- you'll need to think about what you wear if you will be expressing at work (i.e. clothes that undo at the front!)
- bring a spare blouse/shirt with you, in case of leaking milk
- keep a supply of breastpads in your desk
- take a photo of your baby with you, to help trigger the let down reflex
- if you feel a breast leaking, press on your nipple with the heel of your hand
- look after yourself: eat, drink and rest regularly
- remember, more rushing means less milk.

IF YOUR BABY WON'T TAKE A BOTTLE

Don't expect your baby to accept a new feeding method straight away. Introduce a bottle gradually: if you leave plenty of preparation time, you won't feel so pressurised. Some parents have found the following tactics helpful:
- warm up teats to soften them
- try different teats: there are lots of alternatives on the market
- if your baby is old enough, try a beaker
- if your baby is well established on solids, add milk to the food and let her drink water while you are away
- don't offer a bottle in the same feeding position as she is offered the breast
- try to get someone else to give her the bottle-feeds
- offer a bottle when she is calm – not when she is very hungry, for example
- try offering the bottle in a darkened room, so that she does not see it
- if she doesn't take it today, she may do tomorrow. Don't panic.

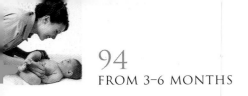
YOUR BED OR HIS COT?

Where your baby sleeps is not a matter of right or wrong. What matters is what's right for you.

From the moment your child is born, you will have to consider two things: the first is how he will feed, and the second is where he will sleep. Both are potentially contentious and friends and family will gather to give you the benefit of their opinions. You may find it useful to listen, and perhaps gain different perspectives. However, the decision is for you and your partner to make alone. It's also useful to be equipped with facts and not just anecdotes.

You'll find it useful to keep an open mind because where your baby sleeps, like how you intend to feed her, doesn't always turn out as planned. You may find that a few sleepless nights and a constantly feeding baby will weaken your resolve to keep your baby out of your bed, for example.

'I always think of later on – if you accept that at some point you will sleep apart, there seems no point in having him in at all. He's happy anyway.'

If you do decide to share your bed with your baby, you'll face different challenges from those that face the parents who opt for a cot. Here is a summary of the main advantages of each choice.

COT SLEEPING MEANS:

• There is no decision to be made about when your baby leaves the family bed. A baby who sleeps alone never gets accustomed to the alternatives.
• Your bedroom remains a place where you can be a couple alone. For many partners, it is vital

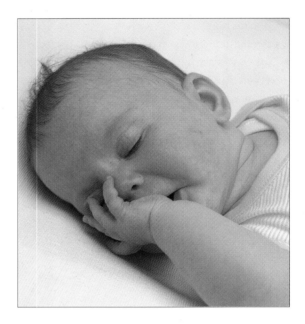

to have a literal space for their relationship. The bedroom is the most obvious choice. It means that they can be alone to make love in peace, or just be together without having that third little person there.
• Everyone has a good night's sleep, not just the baby. For many, the fidgeting and movements of a baby, and later on a toddler, disrupt the night so that parents can't have a peaceful rest. This is more likely to be a problem in later months, as the baby gets older.
• You don't have to worry about rolling onto or otherwise harming your baby. You can have a night out, have a couple of drinks, and not have to worry about the baby being in bed with you.

On the other hand,

CO-SLEEPING MEANS:

• Your baby has easy and immediate access to the breast. If you are breastfeeding, co-sleeping can be very restful, as your baby can feed straight away, and you can doze. This is also a useful method of ensuring a plentiful supply of milk, as she can feed on and off during the night, whilst you barely notice. (You may find you have to check that she is properly latched on in the early days, to avoid soreness.)

'At the moment he is waking up every two to three hours. It doesn't make any sense to get up every time when we can all have a good night's rest.'

• You don't have to keep getting up in the night to check on her. You may find it hard to sleep without checking regularly on your baby, even when she doesn't cry. Having her next to you gives you the security of knowing that she is fine.

• You are doing something you feel is natural. Some parents feel that co-sleeping is in tune with the way humans have developed over thousands of years, giving their children security, plus the benefits of sensory stimuli which, it is argued, aid the child's breathing and development.

For many parents, the main concerns of co-sleeping are whether it increases any risk of cot death, and whether it creates problems in the future, when you will want the child to have a separate bed or cot.

SAFETY FACTORS

Bed-sharing in itself is not a contributory factor in cot death. However, if you share your bed with a baby you should modify your sleeping arrangements, in order to make it as safe as possible for her. If you smoked during pregnancy, or still smoke now, your baby is more at risk when co-sleeping.

YOU SHOULD MAKE SURE THAT:

• Neither of you take any sleeping tablets, alcohol or anything else that makes you drowsy.
• Covers or pillows on the bed cannot overheat your baby, or cover her head.
• There is no heating on in the bedroom during the night and it is well ventilated.
• She is lying on her back.
• The bedroom is smoke-free.

A COMPROMISE?

A middle road is to have her cot or Moses basket in your bedroom. Some cots are made so that they can be attached to the side of the bed. This means you and your baby have easy access to each other while she sleeps separately. You may prefer this.

The best choice, of course, is the one you feel happiest with.

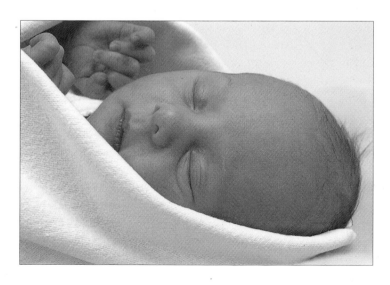

YOUR BABY FROM 6–12 MONTHS

This is when the fun really begins. Your big baby is now strong, confident and responsive. He's ready to take on the world.

By the time he is six months old, you'll start to see the first signs of your baby becoming a person in his own right. He's ready to express what he wants and to try to do something about it. Finally he has escaped the shackles of the reflexes that bound him to certain reactions from the moment he was born. The time has come for him to act spontaneously. Now that his actions are more under his control, he can concentrate for longer, stick with an activity for a few seconds more, and begin to learn about the things going on around him.

Between six months and a year, your baby's memory also takes an upturn. He's beginning to remember things that are repeated and that have some sort of importance for him. For example, around this time your baby will begin to show you that he knows what's coming next at meal-times, bath-times and bed-times. He'll do the same when you tell him favourite rhymes or stories. A few months ago he became excited when he caught sight of the bath or his cot, now he will lean towards (or possibly away from) these familiar experiences.

CRAWLING

Over the next six months your baby will learn to crawl and to pull himself up to standing. Maybe he'll even walk. Crawling provides an example of the way in which the various aspects of a baby's development emerge in parallel. Babies who cannot crawl, don't notice sharp drops or steep slopes (it wouldn't make any difference to them if they did). It's when your baby becomes mobile, that the physical layout of the world suddenly becomes important.

What is amazing is that within a week or two of beginning to crawl, babies eventually learn to stop when they reach the tops of stairs, or slopes that they cannot manage. It's as if their understanding has caught up with their

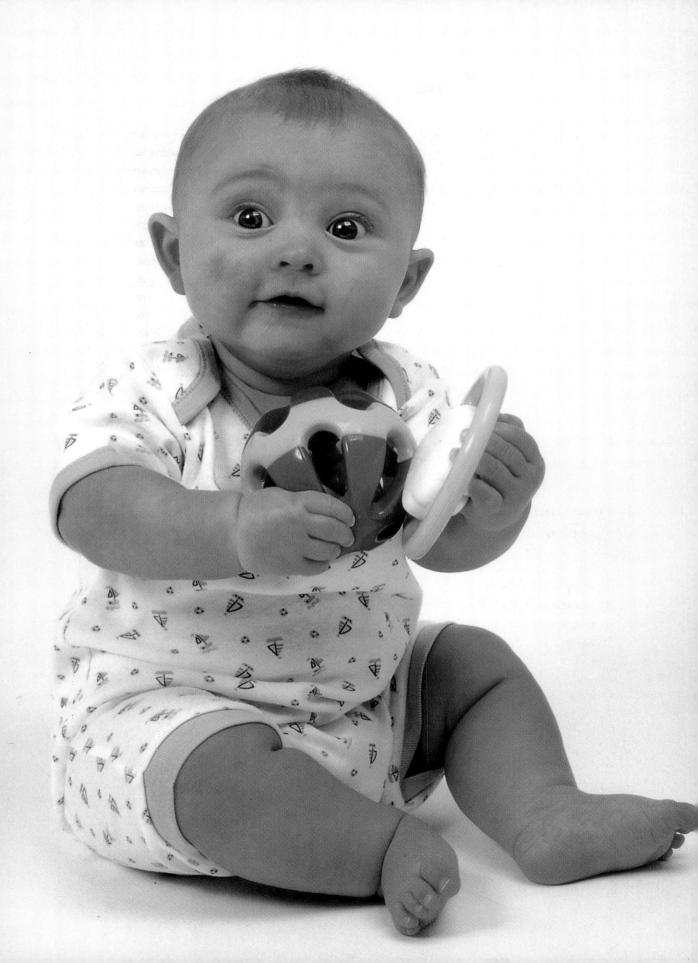

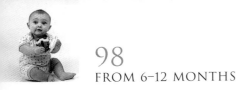
physical development. However, stairgates and a sharp eye are still essential, because babies haven't yet learnt exactly where they start and stop and can accidentally reverse themselves over a drop – even as they turn around to avoid going down it forwards!

Your baby is starting to co-ordinate moving his body with manipulating toys or furniture. By nine months your baby can put together sitting up, reaching and grasping with improved finger control – all of which makes

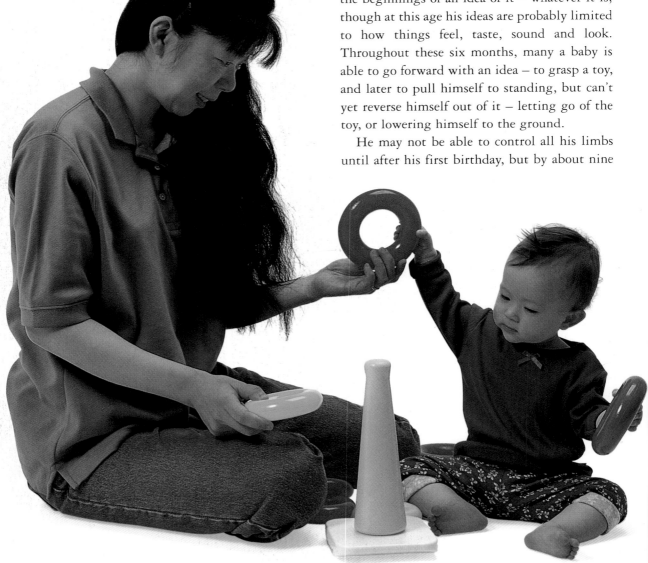

playing more fun, and longer lasting. At this age your baby's mouth is the most sensitive part of his body, so it's no wonder that he uses it so much – anything interesting goes straight to his mouth for exploration.

MAKING PROGRESS

During the second half of your baby's first year he will begin to get a firmer grip on things. Physically, he'll be better able to hold on to anything that he grabs hold of – your hair, a biscuit, the cat – while mentally he'll also have the beginnings of an idea of it – whatever it is, though at this age his ideas are probably limited to how things feel, taste, sound and look. Throughout these six months, many a baby is able to go forward with an idea – to grasp a toy, and later to pull himself to standing, but can't yet reverse himself out of it – letting go of the toy, or lowering himself to the ground.

He may not be able to control all his limbs until after his first birthday, but by about nine

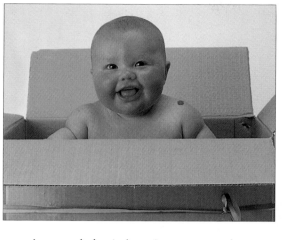

months your baby is learning to control you, and is beginning to do this deliberately, rather than just by accident. When he was little, he would cry and you would go. Now he cries because he wants you to come to him. Now that he knows he has some power over you, he can start to use that power to his advantage. For example, this is when he will keep himself awake deliberately, if he hasn't learnt how to go to sleep easily on his own.

It's probably a good idea to get him used to one or two other important people, just in case, such as a grandmother or childminder as well as yourself and partner, because it's at this stage that he will start to prefer you above all others and become fearful of strangers. Don't be surprised if suddenly he doesn't seem to recognise his Grandma, or he goes all shy with a neighbour he once smiled at. At six months, his memory for faces is not that strong.

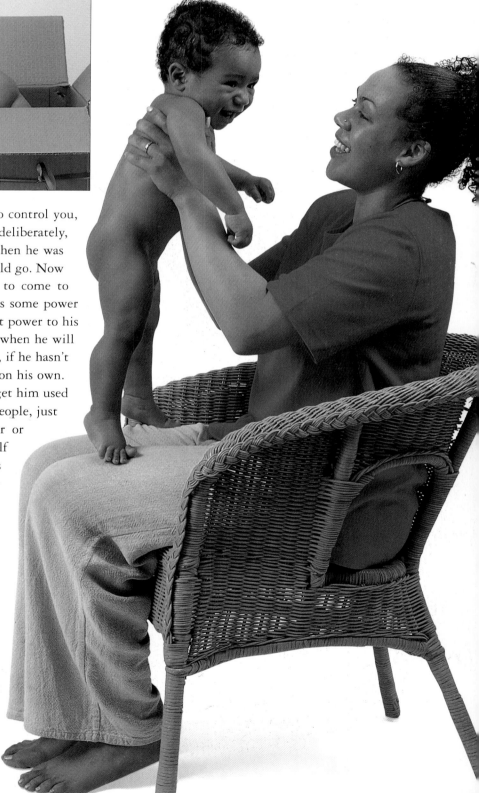

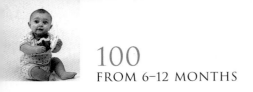

DIARY OF A SIX-MONTH OLD

Paris is six months old. Her parents, Sarah and Peter, both work full-time but they're both able to work at home a couple of days a week, which they combine with looking after Paris. When neither of them is able to work at home, Sarah's mother comes to help out and takes over the care of Paris.

5–6am

Paris wakes up, and plays happily (and noisily) in her cot. Sarah and Peter hear her and take her into their bed for a feed. Until recently, she fell asleep after this feed, but now she stays awake and is very active, kicking and gurgling and grabbing hold of her parents' arms and hair.

'It's wake up and play time,' says Peter. 'It's great fun.'

Depending on who is looking after Paris that day, either Sarah or Peter gets up, leaving the other to play with Paris.

8.30–9am

Sarah or Peter gets Paris up and gives her breakfast. She eats puréed food and likes to try and feed herself, although most of it goes in her hair and her eyebrows and down her clothes. She has her own spoon which she puts into the food, and while she's distracted by that, Sarah or Peter puts a spoonful of food into her mouth. 'When we first started her on solids, she couldn't work out why the food didn't come quickly enough and she screamed,' says Peter. 'So we gave her the spoon to keep her occupied.' They feed her sitting on their laps, so a lot of the food goes over them too. 'Sometimes I take my top off when I feed her,' Sarah says. Paris also has another breastfeed or some expressed breast milk, depending on whether Sarah or Peter is looking after her.

9.30–10am

After breakfast, Paris usually goes into the living room with Sarah or Peter and plays. She can sit unsupported and she especially enjoys sitting in her playnest with her toys around her. She reaches out for a toy, examines it closely – and puts it in her mouth. She also likes to play under her baby gym. She's happy to play on her own, but likes to be able to see Sarah or Peter.

When Paris has had enough of playing with her toys, she puts her arms out to be picked up. Sarah often then takes her out into the garden where they play with the dogs. Paris likes repetitive activities and enjoys it when Sarah throws things for the dogs to fetch. Peter is more likely to play bouncy games with her, standing her on his lap and taking it in turns to blow raspberries, or swinging her in the air.

12–12.30pm

Lunchtime. 'You can tell when she's hungry,' Peter says, 'because she starts getting grizzly.' Lunch is usually puréed vegetables or fruit and breast milk.

1.30pm

After lunch, Paris usually has a nap in her pram or her cot for about half an hour, then it's time for more playing. Occasionally Sarah or Peter takes her out for a walk. Sometimes they try and do household tasks, but these have to be done

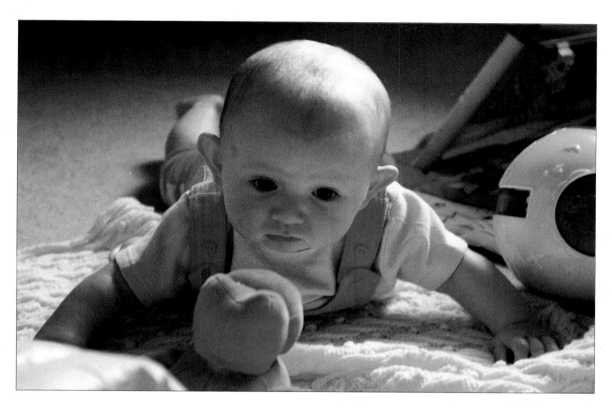

one-handed with Paris sitting on their hip. 'She likes to help,' says Sarah, 'and hates being left out, so the only thing to do is to carry her with you all the time.'

4–5pm

Paris has her tea, again something puréed and some breast milk.

6–7pm

Whichever parent is at work comes home and, says Sarah, 'by that stage you're desperate to hand her over to someone else for a while.' Paris has her bath, which she loves to splash around in, and a breastfeed. Sarah usually gives her a couple of breastfeeds in the evening, not because she's hungry but for comfort.

During the evenings, Paris likes to be with her parents all the time and isn't happy to be left. Sarah and Peter have recently tried putting her in a highchair so that she can be with them while they have their supper. She doesn't like it much, but is delighted with the discovery that you can drop things from it and that someone will pick them up so that she can do it again!

8.30–9.30pm

Paris falls asleep and Sarah or Peter puts her in her cot. She doesn't like to be put in her cot until she's gone to sleep. Once she is asleep she doesn't wake till morning, when, as Sarah puts it, it all starts all over again.

Sarah and Peter find that combining work and looking after Paris as they do isn't always easy, but they feel that it's worth it to be able to spend so much time with her and to have an equal share in her care.

'She's such good fun to be with,' says Peter. 'She's a real delight.'

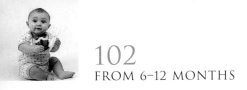

BEGINNING TO TALK

Pointing is one of the earliest ways your baby will try to 'talk' to you and practising making a noise will also start around now.

Communication is a two-way process and depends not only on words but also on facial expressions, gestures and timing. From birth, the feeding process will have taught your baby about taking turns, which is the basis of communication, and since she was a few days old, she will have been tuning in to speech rhythms and eye contact. Now she's ready for some sounds – by six months many babies are making sing-song vowel sounds or single and double 'syllables': a-a, muh, goo, der, or aroo.

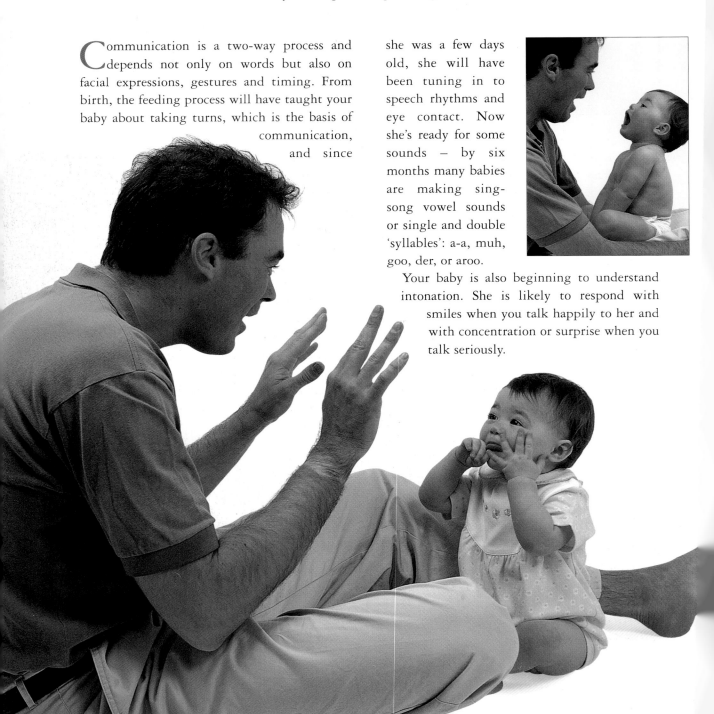

Your baby is also beginning to understand intonation. She is likely to respond with smiles when you talk happily to her and with concentration or surprise when you talk seriously.

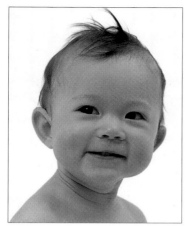 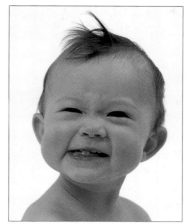 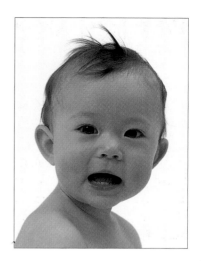

Emily at 10 months watches and imitates funny faces

She's also becoming much more vocal about her likes and dislikes: laughing when a toy does something unexpected or you play peek-a-boo or screaming in annoyance when you refuse to let her feed herself.

UNDERSTANDING 'NO'

By nine months your baby will understand when you say 'no', although it won't always have the effect you'd like. Many babies like to check you're looking their way before they head towards your pot plants or the video. Babies of this age also understand 'bye-bye' and by eight or nine months your baby's wrists will be strong enough for her to wave good-bye from the wrist only. It will be another month or so until she can give a fuller wave.

By now she'll be imitating the sounds you make, and will love doing it. The more that you talk to her, the more she'll babble back loudly and tunefully, using long repetitive strings such as dad-dad-dad and mam-mam. As you talk to her about the car or the latest political scandal, she'll listen and then,

as you stop talking, she'll take her turn by accompanying her babbling with accentuated facial expressions – lots of raised eyebrows, big smiles and head turning. It's the spitting image of you as you talk! She'll also practise her expressive babbling when she's on her own. Even without an audience she still finds it rewarding.

You could start teaching her the words for eyes, nose and mouth – pointing to your own face as you do so. Whether she understands what you're on about or not, she'll still enjoy the game.

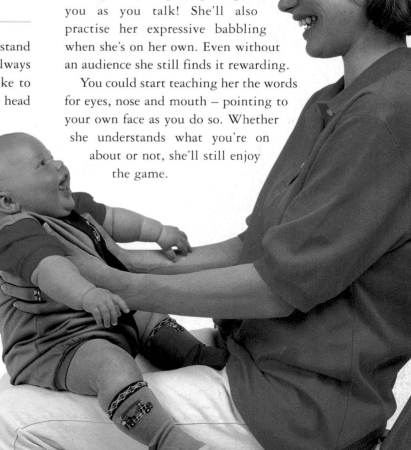

WHAT SHE CAN DO

*Now your baby is starting to reach out and explore her world
eagerly. Everything still goes into the mouth, though, because that
super-sensitive part of the body can teach so much about textures
and taste. Watch out for small things she could choke on.*

At six months a baby is 'visually insatiable',
moving head and eyes in every direction in
an effort to take in the whole of her exciting
world. If you put a toy in front of her, she will
immediately stare at it with interest and, almost
simultaneously, stretch out both hands to grasp
it. At this point, touching and seeing are almost
the same thing for her and both are ways of
gaining information about the world. She'll

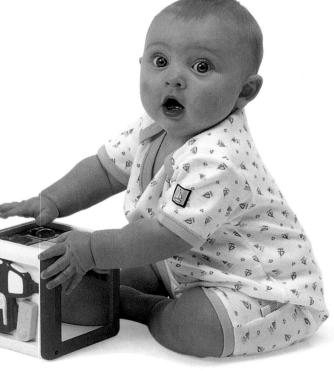

play with your breast
as she feeds, or pat her
bottle as she sucks.

If she's given a toy,
she'll grasp it with
her whole palm and
fingers (called 'palmar
grasp') and pass it
from hand to hand,
now using her hands
as tools rather than
toys in themselves.
She'll also start using
toys as tools, first
banging them together, and then doing things
like dragging a cloth towards her so that
she can reach the toy lying on it.

STRANGER ANXIETY

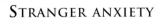

The second half of the first year can be
an emotional time for your baby. At six
months he will probably be friendly
with strangers, but increasingly (from about
seven months) he will be wary, reserved, shy or
anxious if a stranger approaches too nearly or
quickly or when you are out of sight. He's
realising that not everyone is alike, and he
definitely prefers you above all others. He may
hide his face if approached by someone
unfamiliar – in an effort to make them go away!

Within a couple of months the anxiety may
have subsided: 'A couple of months ago, Eleanor
(10$\frac{1}{2}$ months) used to hide her face in my
shoulder, but it's all changed now, in fact she's a
real madam – she'll go to anybody.'

AGE	WHAT CAN SHE DO	TOYS TO PLAY WITH
6 months	Reaches out and grabs one toy at a time with both hands, explores with her mouth, feels with her hands	Towers that you have built for her to knock down Anything safe to go in her mouth and easy to grip
7 to 8 months	Grasps with more control Uses her hands but not fingers Likes to bang two things together Pokes and pulls toys	A saucepan lid and spoon. Two bricks Textured toys with crevices for poking, try chocolate box packaging. Food is good for squishing, and drinks are good for puddling in
7 to 9 months	Passes a toy from hand to hand Points to or pushes tiny things with her forefinger	Toys which look different the other way up – cars, empty yoghurt cartons. Watch and point to the birds in the park or let her push a stumpy crayon around on paper
9 months to 1 year	Can pick things up with a pincer grip (thumb and forefinger) Can let go of toys onto a hard surface	Food is good, especially peas or sweetcorn Put your hand out flat, beneath a toy she is offering you
10 to 11 months	Can let go of toys at will	Drop-the-toy-and-watch-mummy-retrieve-it, becomes a favourite game (It's less tiring for you if you attach her buggy toys to her buggy with short lengths of wool!)

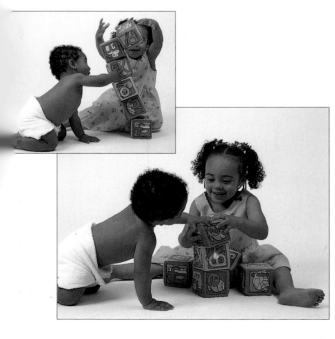

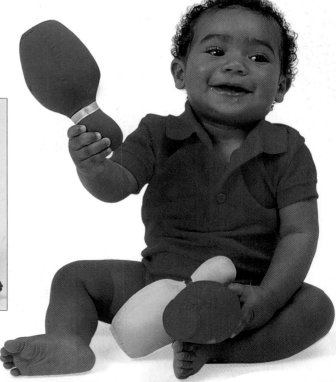

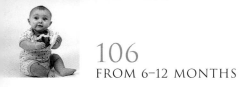
HOW THE WORLD WORKS

Up until about four months, out of sight is out of mind, but by six months your baby will have cottoned on to the idea that things go on being there even when they can't be seen.

If something that your six-month-old is playing with disappears, then he'll look for it. At first, he'll need to be able to see a piece of it poking out but sometime between eight months and a year he'll be able to find his toy even if it rolls completely out of sight, so long as he sees it disappear.

Next time your baby sits in his chair and something falls over the side, watch what he does. He's likely to crane over to watch it fall. This may not look important to you but it is a massive step forward in his development – he's moving his body, eyes and head to track his toy (or the remains of his dinner) because now he knows that even when he can only see part of it the rest is still there. But at this age he still takes things as he finds them – once his toy has fallen on the floor he'll probably forget it.

By nine months your baby is smarter – he knows which direction to look in for a toy, even one which has fallen out of sight. He's on his way to realising that things go on being there even when he can't see them, but he hasn't yet realised that he can make them disappear and reappear. So it will be a few months yet before he'll be ready to play the exciting game of fling-the-teddy-on-the-floor-and-let-mum-pick-him-up!

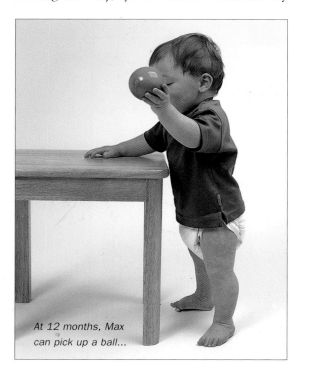

At 12 months, Max can pick up a ball...

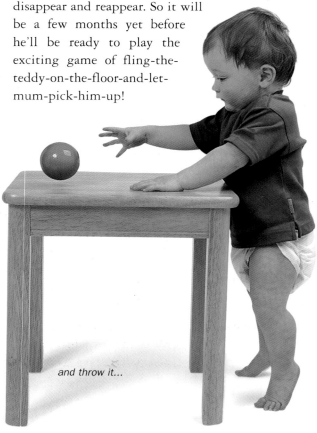

and throw it...

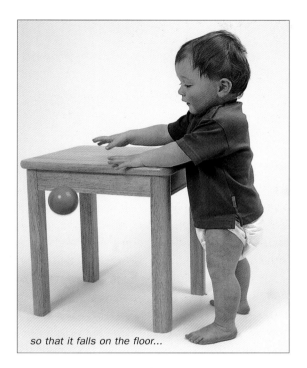

so that it falls on the floor...

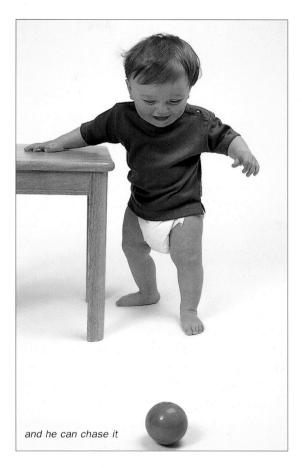

and he can chase it

Meanwhile he'll probably enjoy a few rounds of 'peek-a-boo', in which you take charge of the disappearing and reappearing act. But don't hide for too long or he may get worried. Your baby needs to know you are there right now.

UNDERSTANDING HOW OBJECTS BEHAVE

AGE	STAGE
At birth	She can't see objects as separate from her. If she can't see it, it doesn't exist.
5 months	If an object disappears behind a screen, she will wait to see it come out the other side, but won't be surprised if you switch toys and something completely different comes out.
10 months	She will look for an object where you first hid it, even if she has already seen you move it from that spot. She won't look for an object that she drops.
14 months	Now she will look for something in the right location. She can start to see cause and effect and this means a whole new step forward in play. Her new understanding means that she can start to use tools and plan games.

ROLLING OVER

*If you leave your six-month-old lying on her back, she'll soon try
rolling onto her front. This is the start of getting mobile.*

Your six month old baby is rapidly gaining
control over her upper body, and working
hard to build up her lower body too. At round
about four and a half months she will have
learnt how to
use the weight
of her still
oversized head
to propel
herself from
her front to
her back. The first time she does so may take
you both by surprise, so don't leave her alone on
the changing table.

Rolling from back to front comes later

**'Holly (7 months) turned around
180° on her playmat today. She
was actually trying to roll over,
but the rocking motion swivels
her round rather than over.'**

because lifting your head while lying on your
back takes more effort than raising it while
lying on your front. Try it and see.

Hold her standing and she will bear her
weight on her feet and bounce up and down
vigorously, working out her leg muscles.

If your baby enjoys being upright, try
suspending a baby bouncer from your door and
let her jump for five minutes. Be ready for the
shrieks of laughter as your baby bounces higher
and more vigorously than ever before. If she
enjoys that, you could try putting something
noisy under the bouncer like a big plastic bag
that will make a satisfying racket when your
baby jumps on it.

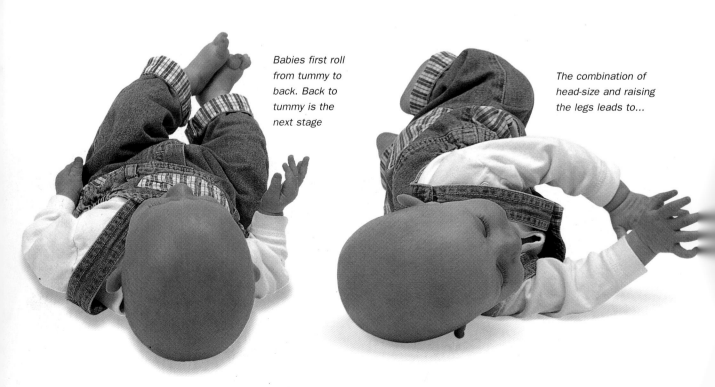

*Babies first roll
from tummy to
back. Back to
tummy is the
next stage*

*The combination of
head-size and raising
the legs leads to...*

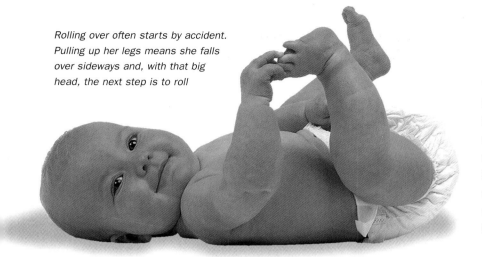

Rolling over often starts by accident. Pulling up her legs means she falls over sideways and, with that big head, the next step is to roll

'The great thing about Bertie (6 months) at the moment is, he can't move! I prop him up on cushions and he's happy to sit and watch me. I'll have my work cut out chasing him once he's mobile.'

Some babies find bouncers alarmingly bouncy, so be guided by their response.

Just before crawling starts, most babies are at their chubbiest. Your child's weight is likely to be pretty high just before she gets mobile. During the second half of a baby's first year, weight-gain slows down considerably as they expend more energy moving around.

You'll also find that a mobile baby needs to wear different clothes. Hardwearing overalls and trousers are practical garments to protect the knees of a crawler. Dresses are out for this stage, except for special occasions, as it's not easy to get around fast in a skirt.

You'll probably also find yourself vacuuming the carpets a lot more frequently when your baby spends most of the time sprawled hands and knees on the floor chewing your rugs!

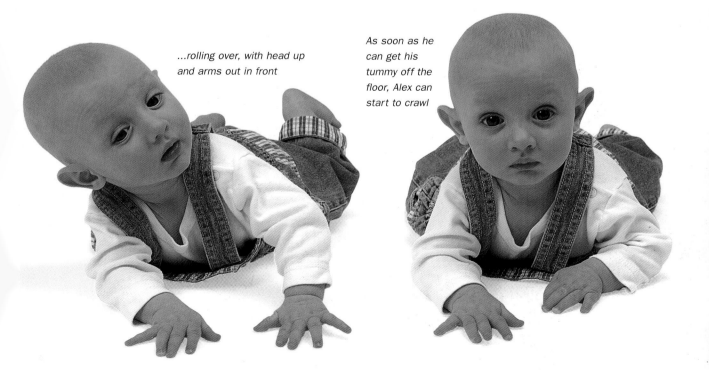

...rolling over, with head up and arms out in front

As soon as he can get his tummy off the floor, Alex can start to crawl

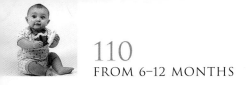

SITTING UP

At the same time as your baby becomes able to sit for longer she becomes fascinated by what happens to things when she strokes, pokes, prods and pulls them.

Your baby will want to sit up, but until about nine months he won't be able to get himself into that position. It's your job to help him get there so that he can practise balancing. By six months he will probably be able to sit unsupported for just a few seconds, with his head erect and his back straight, but he'll soon topple over, so support him well with cushions on all sides.

By eight months his back will be strong enough and he will have enough control to sit unsupported for longer without the cushions for help (but do leave them in a circle around him for when his balancing act ends).

By nine or ten months he will be able to sit alone on the floor for ten to fifteen minutes, but the cushions can still offer him a more comfortable way down.

Don't leave him sitting alone until he is able to get himself into and out of a sitting position – if he fell over face down he could smother himself.

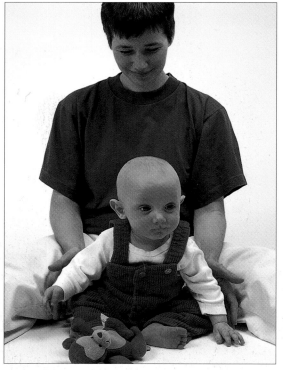 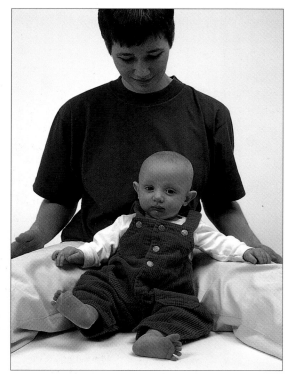

Alex, aged 5 months, still needs a little help from Mum if he is to sit up without toppling over

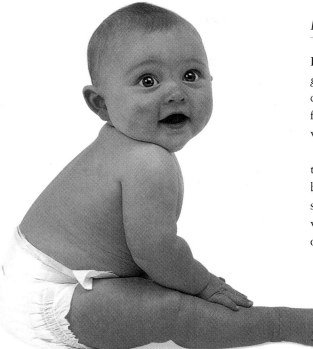

At 6 months, Luke can sit up but not hold his back straight yet. It's an effort to play for long in this position.

MUSCLE CONTROL

Brain development is going on as your baby grows, meaning that brain cells are making connections which control and exercise muscles from the top of the body downwards, starting with the muscles of the face.

Gradually, the area of the brain that controls the neck, shoulders and back develops, followed by arms, hands and fingers. Control of the legs starts with hips, then moves to legs and feet, which is why walking doesn't start until the end of the first year.

SITTING-UP PLAY

Once sitting has been mastered, your baby will want to get hold of everything and explore it! Cats, cushions, cornflakes and carpets may all receive fond attention. She no longer likes to just grab and mouth things as she did when she was younger. Now she wants to examine them in all their potential – and her hands are much better for this. It's taken her a long time to learn how to hold onto things, and it'll take her until she's about ten months old to learn how to let go of them.

Emily, at 10 months, has a straight back and is perfectly comfortable manipulating toys

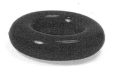

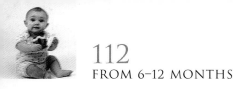

GETTING MOBILE

Your baby will need a lot of practice before he can crawl. Put him on the floor as often as you can, with a few toys just out of reach, and watch him move.

At around about six months your baby will make his first attempts to crawl – pulling his legs up beneath him while lying on his tummy, and pushing up with his hands. But that's all he'll manage – a crawling position, without the crawl! And for the next couple of months it'll be the same story – top marks for effort, but none at all for movement.

By about nine months your baby will spend most of his time poised for take-off in true crawling style, rocking backwards and forwards, raring to go but still without moving. He may squirm or roll his way across the floor in desperation, but without any control over where he ends up.

Between nine and ten months most babies finally start to move – but sometimes backwards. He wants to go forwards, he's trying to go forwards, but his arms are stronger than his legs, and he ends up further away from the interesting object he's seen, rather than closer.

CRAWLING STYLES

Most babies learn to crawl on their hands and knees, but some prefer to walk like bears on their hands and feet, which looks funny but is often just as fast. A few lie flat on their tummies and pull themselves along with their arms, which are still stronger than their legs – commando-style – and others (usually early sitters) learn to

'Now that she's learnt to crawl Eleanor (at 10 months) likes to get hold of the newspaper – the Sports section – lie on her back and rip it to shreds. She gets covered in newsprint: the other day I could read her left cheek!'

Emily has her own crawling style – a half-and-half bottom-shuffle involving one foot and the other knee

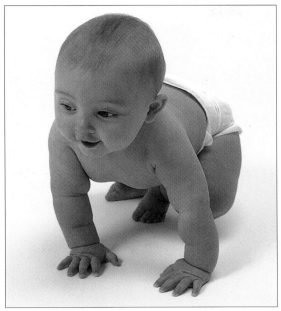

Instead of getting onto his knees...

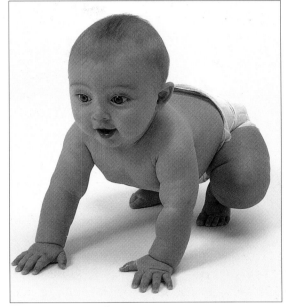

Luke goes onto his feet

bottom-shuffle, and go straight from here to pulling themselves up, missing out conventional crawling altogether. It's entirely a matter of preference, and each method is as good as the rest, although bottom-shufflers and commandos often walk later.

When he is up to speed a crawling baby can reach two kilometres an hour, and may cover around 200 metres a day. This means you'll now need to have 'eyes in the back of your head' to make sure he doesn't have an accident. See 'Making your home safe' overleaf.

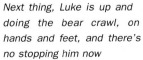

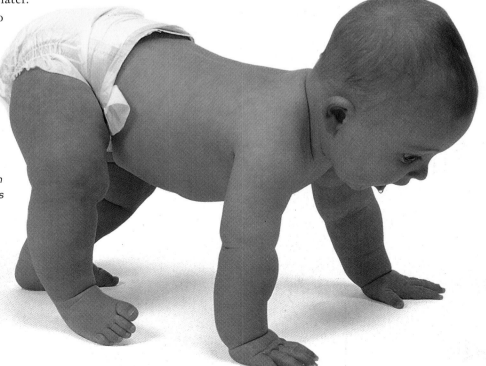

Next thing, Luke is up and doing the bear crawl, on hands and feet, and there's no stopping him now

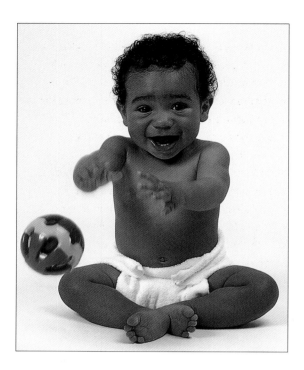

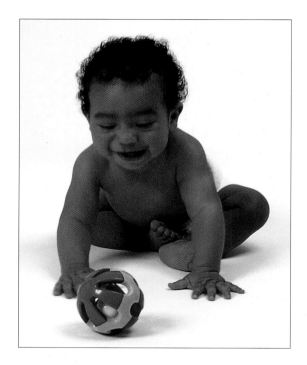

KEEP IT OUT OF REACH

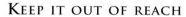

Don't rely on childproof packaging or safety catches. Put the following items well out of reach on a high shelf or cupboard:

- medicines
- alcohol
- cleaning materials
- beauty products
- cigarettes, lighters and ashtrays
- matches
- anything hot
- sharp implements (cutlery, tools, sewing equipment, razors)
- anything small enough to swallow
- any breakables and heavy ornaments
- jewellery
- plastic bags and cling-film
- disposable nappies – if she chews them she could choke on the wadding
- heavy books – she could pull them off the shelf on top of herself
- older children's toys
- plants – they could be poisonous.

Some things are less conveniently stored at a high level, but still need to be kept away from your baby. This includes rubbish bins – just imagine – and pet food bowls.

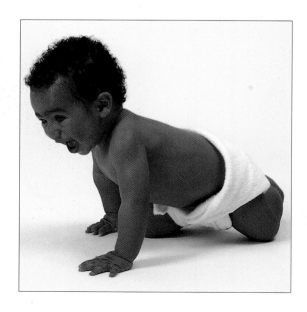

MAKING YOUR HOME SAFE

When your baby starts to crawl and to pull herself up to a standing position, you'll quickly realise that your perfectly ordinary home is in fact a minefield. Innocent objects take on a new significance as you realise what your baby can do with them. The best way of preventing accidents is never to leave your baby unattended – not while you answer the phone or the door, or even when you go to the loo. Take her with you or put her in a playpen. Also, follow these simple safety tips:

- fit a stairgate at the bottom and the top of your stairs
- put guards in front of fires and hot radiators
- put socket covers on empty electrical sockets
- switch electrical appliances off at the wall
- fix a cooker guard round your hob
- fit safety catches to any drawers, cupboards or windows that your baby can reach
- use locks for your fridge, freezer, washing machine and tumble drier
- make sure you don't leave any trailing leads anywhere, especially on your kettle or iron
- don't leave your ironing board and iron out
- use safety glass or safety film over low glass
- put tablecloths, unstable furniture, and glass-topped tables away until your baby is older
- fit smoke detectors on every level of your house, and buy a fire extinguisher.

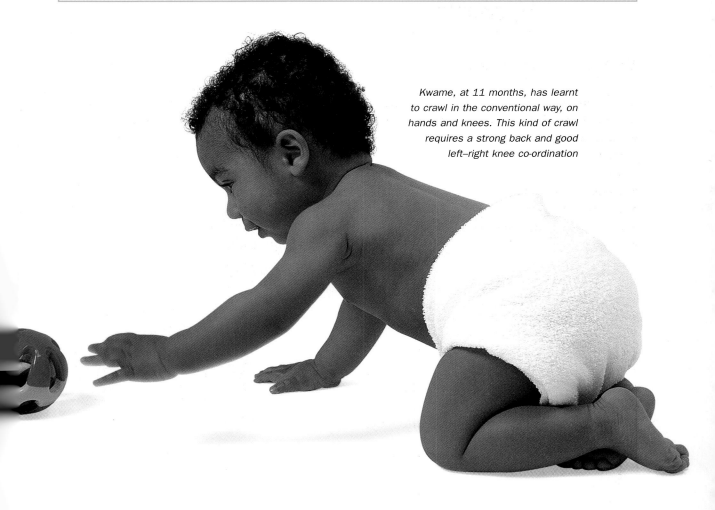

Kwame, at 11 months, has learnt to crawl in the conventional way, on hands and knees. This kind of crawl requires a strong back and good left–right knee co-ordination

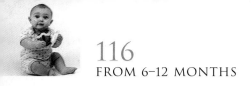
TEETHING

You can expect your baby to get his first tooth at sometime around six months, although it can happen earlier – it's also not unknown for babies of a year to have no teeth.

Some babies seem to cut teeth without any trouble at all, while for others it can be a long and distressing process, lasting for weeks. The normal symptoms of teething are dribbling and wanting to gnaw or chew on something, often accompanied by grizzling and fretfulness and sometimes by red cheeks. But although teething can make your baby uncomfortable and grumpy, it doesn't make him ill. If he's off his food, or is vomiting, or has diarrhoea or a fever, the cause is something else and you should consult your doctor or health visitor.

All babies' teeth come through in the same order, although at different times for different babies, starting with the lower front ones. If you think your baby might be teething, check his bottom gum to see if it looks at all inflamed. If there's a little pale bump in the middle of the gum, it'll probably be followed in a few days by a small sharp tooth.

Give your children plain water to drink from an early age and they won't get a taste for tooth-destroying flavoured, fizzy drinks when they're older

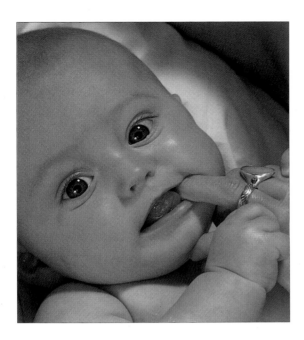

How can i help?

If teething is proving to be an uncomfortable and distressing process for your baby, you'll want to do whatever you can to help. Try these suggestions:

• Rub his gums gently with your (clean) finger.
• Give him something hard to chew on, like a raw carrot, a hard rusk, or a teething ring. These may be more soothing if they've been chilled for a while in the fridge.
• Teething gels, which contain anaesthetics, can be helpful, especially if the discomfort is keeping him awake at night, but their effect is short-lived and they cause allergies in some babies.
• If the soreness is stopping him from sleeping, some paracetamol syrup can help, but try not to use it too frequently.
• Don't take him out in cold weather. If you can't avoid going out, wrap his head and face in a warm hat and scarf.
• Give him lots of cuddles.

Caring for your baby's teeth

First teeth are very small, but they still need to be cleaned every day. You can do this by rubbing the teeth with a clean finger or clean handkerchief or piece of gauze or cotton bud with baby toothpaste on it, or you can use a baby toothbrush. Some babies enjoy playing with a toothbrush and waving it around in their mouths, but although this may be a first step towards brushing their own teeth, it's not a substitute for adult brushing.

Using a fluoride toothpaste can help prevent tooth decay, though check the packaging to make sure that it doesn't contain any sugar. Some dentists recommend giving children fluoride supplements as well, but in many areas fluoride is added to the water supply, and giving extra fluoride on top of that can cause discolouration in the teeth. Before giving your baby any supplements, therefore, check with your dentist what the situation is in your area.

FEEDING A BABY WITH TEETH

• There's no need to stop breastfeeding just because your baby has a tooth. Some mothers continue breastfeeding till their child is over two, by which time he will have almost a complete set of teeth. If he does bite when he's breastfeeding, draw him towards the breast so that his nose is blocked and he has to let go to breathe.
• Give him plenty of hard foods to chew on.
• Avoid sweet sugary foods and drink.
• For healthy teeth, your baby needs calcium (found in milk, cheese, yoghurt) and vitamin D (found in egg yolk and fatty fish, like sardines). If your baby dislikes any of these, ask your health visitor for advice.

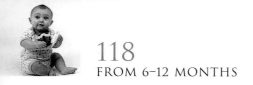

FIRST FOODS

Your baby will thrive on breast milk alone for at least the first four months of her life, and if you prefer, you can leave weaning until she is six months. After that, she'll need more to nourish her than milk alone.

If you start your baby on solids too soon (before she's four months old) her digestive system may not be sufficiently developed, and this may make her more susceptible to allergies and food intolerances. Since milk is a complete food at this stage, adding solids to her diet will mean she has less room for what she needs: milk.

'I was dreading the mess, but it wasn't as bad as I thought it would be.'

And leaving weaning beyond six months may result in a baby who is reluctant to adapt to the different textures and tastes of solid foods. Your baby also needs more iron in her diet than either breast or bottled milk contains, as her own supplies will be running low by now.

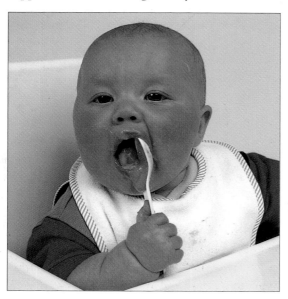

THE BEST TIME FOR YOUR BABY?

Look out for:
- a growing interest in your food
- a return to more disturbed nights
- hungrier during the day.

If any of these happen before you want to start on solids, you could increase the amount of milk that she has. If you are breastfeeding, letting her feed on demand means that she will increase the milk supply by herself over a day or two.

HOME MADE OR COMMERCIAL?

Babies can enjoy both types of food. It is certainly cheaper to prepare your own baby food, and, as long as there is no added salt or other additives, it's easy to take your baby's vegetable portion after it has been cooked with the rest of the family's and just mash it up or purée it. Alternatively, you can cook a larger amount of fruit or vegetables and freeze portions in sterilised ice-cube trays, ready to defrost small amounts for your baby's meal.

'I made a wonderful meal, and the whole lot came back.'

Many parents find the convenience of commercially prepared food useful if they have a busy schedule. If you use jars of baby food, remember to read the labels to check the ingredients. At this early stage, your baby needs no additives or sugar in food. Many of the fruit purées, such as banana or peach, are very sweet anyway. Adding sugar only develops a taste for more.

GETTING STARTED

A good time to start offering your baby solid food is when it is sandwiched between two milk feeds. So at her feed time, just offer half her usual amount of milk. This means the edge will have been taken off her hunger, but she won't be too full. Then she can finish off with more milk after eating.

At this stage, don't expect your baby to be taking very much food: one or two teaspoons will be enough at the beginning. She will also need to get used to the technique of eating with a spoon. Remember, this is very different from what she is used to, and at first, she will probably push out more than she takes in.

It's a good idea to introduce new foods one at a time, particularly if you have a family history of allergies.

Try either feeding her on your lap, or putting her in a bouncy chair in front of you to feed, as she probably won't be ready to sit in a high chair yet. This will be a messy business – keep a damp cloth and plenty of bibs handy.

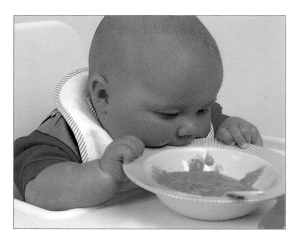

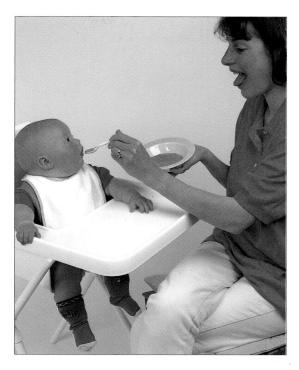

STARTER FOOD

The first solid foods that your baby has should be simple: mashed or puréed vegetables and fruit, and baby rice to add bulk. If you want, you can mix the baby rice with expressed breast milk or formula milk, or with the fruit or vegetables.

Experiment with tastes and textures, particularly as she grows older. Whilst first foods should be as smooth and liquid as possible, gradually make the texture coarser as the weeks go by. Offer a variety of foods, and if she doesn't like something one day, she may eat it happily the next; you can always try again. You can also disguise the taste of something by adding it to one of her favourites.

Foods to avoid: salt, sugar and nuts. Gluten (contained in wheat, rye, barley and oats), citrus fruits, meat and fish for the first six months. Eggs, cow's milk and spices for the first year.

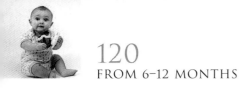

CHANGING A MOBILE BABY

'Basically, it's a struggle,' is what one dad had to say about changing a wriggling baby's nappy.

Once your baby has gained a degree of control of his body and limbs, and even more so once he can crawl, his response to being placed on his back to have his nappy changed may well be like that of an upturned beetle – he will do all he can to get himself the right way up again. This makes nappy-changing rather more difficult than when he was younger.

Fortunately, as he gets older, your baby won't need to have his nappy changed as frequently as he did when he was tiny. He may well only have one dirty nappy a day, and, as his bladder gets bigger and able to hold more urine, he'll have fewer wet ones.

There are various things you can try to help minimise the nappy-changing struggle:

• Give your baby a toy to hold. This may distract him, especially if it's one that makes a noise, and it will help keep his hands away from the nappy area. It doesn't always work though, as Helen found: 'If I give him a toy, he just throws it down in disgust.'

• If you always change him in the same place, have a mobile for him to look at. He'll probably try to reach out and grab hold of it, so make sure it's out of his range or securely fixed.

• Play a musical box, or a tape, or sing to him.

• Make funny faces and blow raspberries at him to hold his attention.

• Play tickling games.

• Put him in clothes that are easily removed, so that you can be as quick as possible.

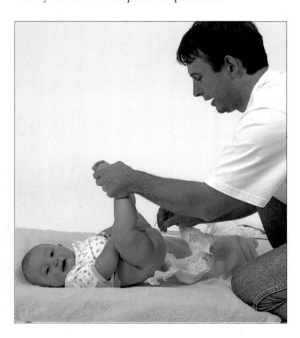

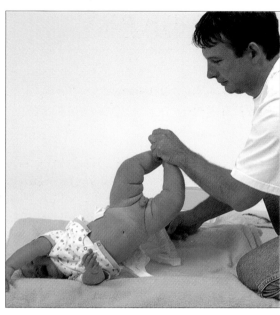

Changing a mobile baby can be a race against time. Try blowing raspberries or making faces to hold his attention!

always easy to put it on straight. If you try to change your baby standing up once he can walk, he is, of course, quite likely to toddle off in the middle of it.

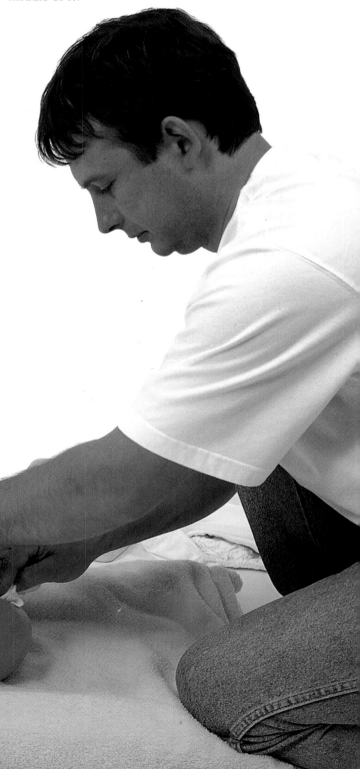

• Change him on your lap. Not everyone finds this easy, but for some parents, like Lucy, it's the only way they can get the nappy changed. 'I have her on my lap, put my arm across her chest to hold her down, and change the nappy as quickly as I can.'
• If he's able to, let him stand up and hold on to something while you change him. The holding on will keep his hands occupied. It's easier to put a disposable or a shaped cloth nappy on like this than a folded terry, and it isn't

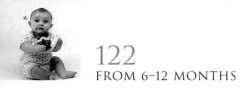

BATHING YOUR OLDER BABY

Once your baby is eating solid food and crawling around on the floor, you'll probably find that by the end of the day, she's pretty grubby and will need a bath.

Fortunately, most older babies enjoy being bathed and you may well want to give your baby a daily bath, whether she's grubby or not. As well as being fun, bathtime has the merit of being relaxing too, and it can form part of a regular evening wind-down routine in readiness for bed.

By the age of six months, most babies will have outgrown their baby bath, and if they haven't, they'll probably be kicking and splashing in it so much that you'll emerge from bathtime as if you've just been in the bath yourself. But no matter how much they've enjoyed the baby bath, some babies are rather frightened of going into an adult-sized bath at first. To help ease the transition, you can try putting the baby bath inside the ordinary one for a few days until your baby gets used to it.

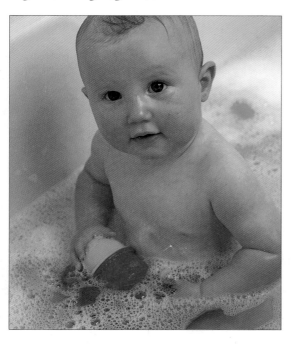

• Get everything that you need together (towel, toiletries, bath toys, changing mat, nappy, clothes) before you start – and put it all where you can reach it with one hand (though keep the obvious things well out of splashing range so they don't get soaked).

• Fill the bath to the depth of about 10–13cm. Put the cold in first, then add the hot. As when you were using the baby bath, test the water temperature with your elbow – it should feel pleasantly warm – or with a bath thermometer.

• Add some baby bath liquid if you want to. You may want to avoid it if you know your baby's skin is especially sensitive.

• Undress her and lift her into the bath. If she can't yet sit unsupported, you'll need to support her back with your arm round her shoulders and your hand under her armpit. It's better for your back if you kneel by the bath rather than bending over it. Some parents use a bath support or bath seat for their baby, which leaves both their hands free for washing and playing with the baby.

• Wash her with your free hand or with a flannel or sponge. If you use a flannel or sponge, you'll probably find that she'll try to grab it, so you might like to give her one of her own to hold while you wash her. If you do, it'll go straight into her mouth, of course, so it might be better to hold off on the bath liquid otherwise she'll be getting that in her mouth too. A lot of babies don't like water on their faces, so make sure you squeeze the flannel out before washing her face (once your baby gets to about six months you no longer need to use boiled water for this). And keep soap or bath liquid away from her eyes and mouth.

• Baths are as much for playing in as for getting clean in, so give her lots of playing time. She'll probably like toys that float, or from which water can be poured or squeezed or squirted, or which have holes in them that the water can run through. If your bath has a shower attachment, she may like playing with that too, but make sure the water isn't too hot.

• Take her out before the water becomes too cold, even though she'll probably protest loudly. Lift her out by holding her under both armpits – she'll be slippery – and wrap her in a towel.

Some parents enjoy having a bath with their baby. Says Andrew, 'Jack and I have a great time splashing around and pouring water over each other.'

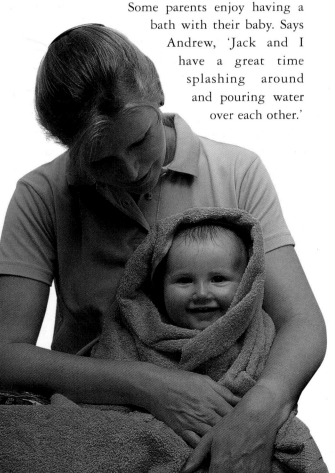

HAIRWASHING

Although most older babies enjoy being in the bath, a lot of them hate having their hair washed. If yours is one who does, you'll probably want to keep hairwashing to a minimum – quite a lot can be accomplished just by gentle brushing and by rubbing over her hair with a damp flannel.

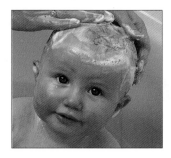

When you have to wash her hair, a shampoo shield can help. If that doesn't work, you can try washing her hair before you put her in the bath.

The easiest way is probably to have a bowl of water on the bathroom floor, and to kneel next to it, with your baby lying on her back on your lap, with her head over the bowl. If you wet – and rinse – her hair with a flannel, you won't get any water in her eyes. Give her a toy to hold to keep her occupied and you're less likely to have to cope with waving arms getting in the way.

BATHTIME SAFETY

• Never leave your baby unattended in the bath. If the phone rings, or the doorbell goes, ignore it. If you find you've forgotten something, do without it or wait till you've got her out of the bath before you go and get it.

• A rubber mat in the bottom of the bath can make it less slippy.

• Don't add hot water to the bath while your baby is in it.

• If the hot tap feels hot after you've run the water, wrap a flannel round it.

• Don't let her pull herself up on the side of the bath.

• Keep any soap or bath liquid or shampoo out of your baby's reach.

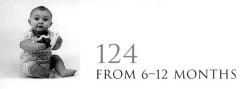

BEDTIME ROUTINES

The common way of marking the transition between day and night is to set up a routine, which leads to bedtime. For parents, this means that they can look forward to having some time together alone.

A soothing going-to-bed routine can be very comforting for a baby. If it comes at the same time every day, she will even look forward to this special time of being pampered by you before the separation of sleep.

You will also look forward to time alone after a demanding day with your baby – something that may be even more important for single parents, who need to have evenings when they can be themselves at last and relax, baby-free, for a while.

CHANGING FROM DAY TO NIGHT

Your baby will learn that the mood will change from activity to rest, from noise to peacefulness, from stimulation to relaxation towards the end of the day. An evening routine can slow her pace down.

'For your own sanity, it helps to have a routine. By 8.30pm, we can sometimes have a life of our own.'

As your winding-down routine starts to keep to a pattern, so she will learn that one thing follows another. You will both be tired, but try to make it a positive end to the day.

Many routines start with the last meal of the day, followed by a bath. Whilst your baby is unlikely to need a bath every night, it can be pleasant to spend half an hour in quiet play with her. A soak in warm water can be very relaxing, and you could always take a dip with her

yourself. (Make sure you can get her in and out of the bath safely if you are alone.)

If you don't want to bath her every night, then giving her a top and tail, changing her nappy and putting her into a nightsuit will be just as good.

Once she's freshened up and in nightclothes, choose a quiet activity, such as sitting together and looking at a book

'I'd rather he was awake when he goes into his cot, but sometimes he just drops off on the breast.'

while having a cuddle. Then let her hold a special teddy or soft toy while you sing a few lullabyes. She can hang on to the teddy when you depart.

A LAST FEED AND...

Babies do need help to get to sleep, but ultimately, if you want your baby to drift off to sleep alone, you just have to let her practise. If you put her in her cot and stay with her, singing, stroking and comforting her, she may need you to do this for her every time she wakes up.

Many babies will wake as the sun rises, and expect you to be as lively as they are. Make sure their room is full of bright colours and pictures, so that there's plenty to look at when they wake up. Put toys in the bottom of the cot, and cloth books, too. You could gain precious minutes of sleep this way!

'WITH A LITTLE BIT OF HELP'...

While babies love the comfort of a pair of arms, a warm breast or a bottle, there are ways in which they can learn to comfort themselves. Some of these are:

- Thumb-sucking. Love it or hate it, some babies are just thumb-suckers, and at sleep time, this can be a useful habit. Thumbs don't get lost in the way that dummies do.
- Dummy/comforter. The up-side of giving your baby a dummy is that, when you want her to give it up, you can remove it. (Hardly likely in the case of thumbs.)
- Favourite toy/blanket. If you give her a cloth or article of clothing which has your smell on it, she can hold it while feeding. Then when on her own, she should derive comfort from it. These objects of affection tend to last for a few years, and are likely to travel with your baby everywhere – so make sure it's nothing too embarrassing.
- Musical mobile. A wind-up mobile can be great company as you leave the room, but can often (unfortunately) mean that you have to keep coming back to re-wind.
- A night-time light show. You can get lamps for baby bedrooms that throw a delightful kaleidoscope of colours on to the ceiling for your sleepy baby to enjoy.
- Ask your health visitor for help if necessary.

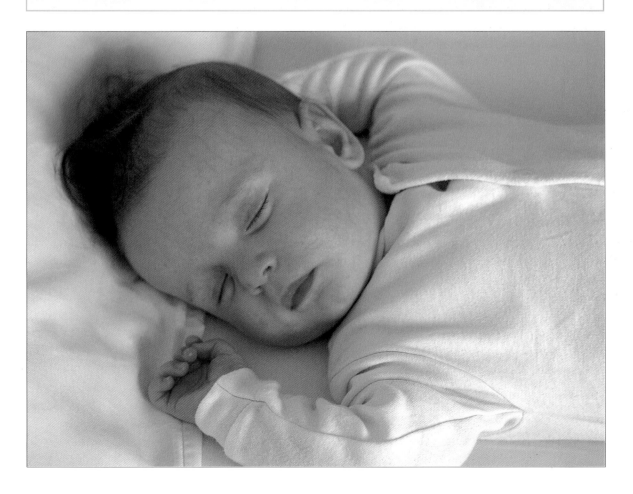

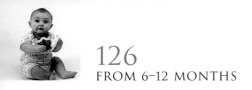
TRANSITION TO PARENTHOOD

'I think that I felt I was really a parent when I had learnt that you're not going to get everything right, but you will survive anyway. I understand what "good enough parenting" means. Sometimes that's all you can do.'

It's often not until your baby is six to twelve months old that you can really sit back and begin to feel that you are getting to grips with the job of being a parent. Everyone who has ever experienced it, says nothing can really prepare you for the huge upheaval, both physical and emotional, that a new baby brings to their lives. By the second half of the first year, however, things should be starting to settle down and you should feel more in charge.

The birth of a baby changes the relationship between a couple forever. Whilst it can be enhancing, there are many things about this time in life that can create stress. For example, lack of sleep for weeks and sometimes months on end can leave parents ragged and irritable, particularly if they are unsure why their baby does not sleep so well. Lack of experience can make parents feel defensive, and often critical of the other partner. A problem such as colic can put rationalism to the test, taking worn out parents to the limit of their tolerance. Add to this a household that may be experiencing a cash-flow shortage due to one partner stopping work, or paying childcare costs, and it's easy to see how communication can break down.

A new baby obviously needs an enormous amount of nurture from his mother. This puts a huge demand on you and means you'll want more love and attention, in turn, from your partner. On the other hand, he's deprived of your usual emotional support during this time, and if he just can't cope with a lot less cherishing than he's used to, he can't help you when you most need it.

It can be helpful to think of your ability to give endless love and affection as an 'emotional storecupboard' that needs constant stocking up if you are to draw from its supplies. No one can really give love unless they're getting it, too.

It's important to tell each other what you want. Don't expect your partner to read your mind. Try to be clear and honest.

When you have important things to talk over, try to pick the right time and be aware of your feelings. Stick to 'I' phrases, such as 'I feel lonely' rather than 'you' phrases like 'you're never here'. Be prepared to negotiate, and agree to differ – don't always insist on having the last word. Caresses help a lot, too: whether given or received, the effect seems to be the same. Be hands-on loving.

Sometimes partners need lessons in 'relationship skills', such as negotiating, communicating, expressing affection and doing their share. Many of us didn't learn these skills in our own families, but they're vital.

Think of your relationship as the root out of which the whole structure of your new life needs to grow and flourish. Keep talking, spending time together, listening to each other, considering each other. You depend on each other and should take care of each other.

This is a time, if you haven't done so already,

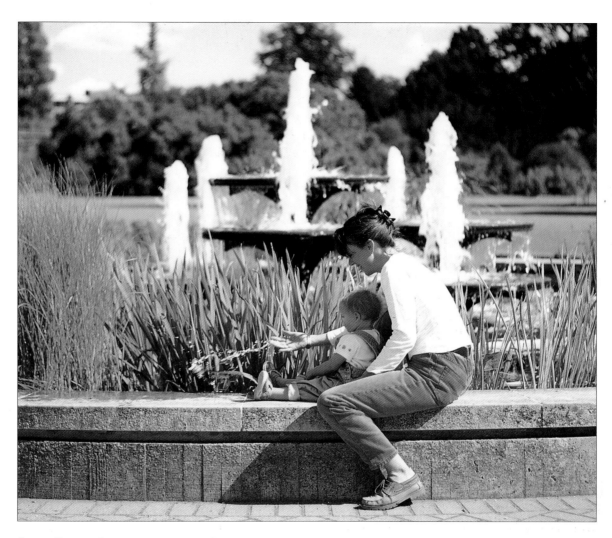

for talking about your past, finding what experiences you have in common, what you feel about certain important issues, such as discipline, smacking, sleep arrangements. You may be surprised to find that your partner has very different views from you about how to bring up children, and these differences will be worth exploring together.

PHYSICAL CHANGES

So there is emotional change in your relationship to adapt to, but you will also be

coping with the day to day work of being a parent. At times this is sheer physical hard work. Babies, pushchairs and car seats are all heavy, and regularly need moving. By the time your baby is a year old, you will still need to do a lot of this physical work, whilst the baby gets bigger and bigger. Also, the time for relaxing is often snatched away from us by the demands of a baby who doesn't understand that mummy hasn't sat down all day.

'I am staggered by how much carrying and lifting I do as a mother.'

On the other hand, the picture of parenthood

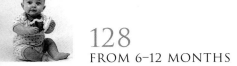

also has many positive aspects to recommend it.

By the time your baby reaches her first birthday, your roles as parents are likely to be well defined. Your status within the family may have changed. Many women say that their parents treat them as adults for the first time once they have children. It is as though they have joined the parents' club.

As a daughter becomes aware, through her own experience as a mother, of how much love, worry and effort is involved in caring for a baby, she often sees her mother with different eyes, appreciating her as she couldn't before the arrival of children. On the other hand, disagreements over babycare or unwelcome attempts to encroach on the new parents' territory can make this relationship a tricky one.

Fathers, too, will begin to think a lot more about the past. The way that they themselves were fathered will begin to influence the way they now care for the baby, either following the model of their parents or deciding to do things differently.

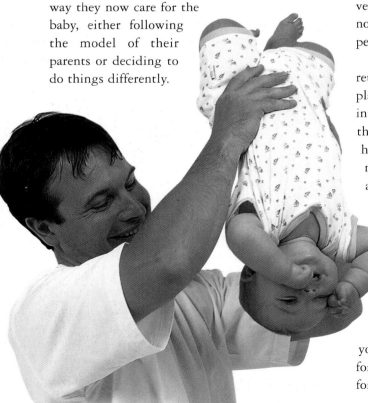

Fortunately, as new parents, you are not destined to repeat the old patterns. In fact, the more you can understand your relationship with your own parents, and come to terms with it, the less likely you are to repeat it.

It can be a difficult and poignant time for parents who themselves experienced an unhappy childhood. If this is the case for you or your partner, try to talk it through and learn from it.

BACK TO WORK

Sometimes it's a relief to get back to work outside the home and rediscover the self you were before you had a baby, even though this will add to your busy schedule. In fact, you'll probably find that you've never worked as hard in your life before and that being a working mum stretches your organisational skills to the very limit. But there will be rewards, too, and not just financial ones – such as meeting new people and using your career talents.

Good childcare is the key to a successful return to work, and you'd be wise to start planning well in advance. Provision of childcare in Britain isn't perfect – during your search for the right set-up, you're likely to find things hampered by childminders with no vacancies, nurseries that don't meet your expectations, and nannies you wouldn't feel happy to leave your child with. But at least choice in childcare is improving – see over the page for more information.

The decision to return to work doesn't just involve practical changes – it will also involve an emotional upheaval during which you'll almost certainly re-prioritise what matters most in your life. Give it careful thought – what works for other people might not be the right solution for you and your partner.

BREASTFEEDING AT SIX MONTHS

Breastfeeding a sturdy six-month-old is a pleasure shared. You'll find it easy, especially as your baby will have started solids, and you won't have the problem of extra equipment to clean, sterilise and transport. It's also easy to breastfeed out and about.

Many women plan to stop breastfeeding at six months and move on to bottles. While it is perfectly normal, on a global scale, to continue breastfeeding well into the second year, women in the western world do tend to wean earlier than that. Obviously, you must do what feels comfortable for you and your baby, and make a choice that fits in with your current lifestyle. You may long to get your body back and want to stop, or you may enjoy the ease of breastfeeding now and decide to carry on.

Some women choose to continue to breastfeed for another six months: 'Now I've got this far, I might as well carry on for a year rather than use formula and bottles and have to sterilise for six months.' Your baby can start using a beaker with a spout, at this stage, for mid-day drinks of juice or water and you won't need to worry about getting him used to a bottle after the breast.

However, a six-month-old is far more aware of surroundings and stimulus than a new baby and can easily be distracted from the breast when other activities are going on. 'He would latch on, then something would grab his attention and he'd turn his head quickly. Unfortunately, my nipple would still be in his mouth!'

This can be a trying time for the breastfeeding mother, as well as being painful and frustrating. It doesn't tend to last long, though, and he should relax back again into settled feeding. In the meantime, you may find it useful to go into a quiet room for feeds. Remember too, that all the time he is getting more proficient at feeding, and can take most of his feed very quickly.

The arrival of first teeth can occasionally result in a baby chewing, or biting on the breast. This is very painful and you're likely to shout or scream. But this reaction can cause delight in the baby, unaware of the pain caused, but pleased that his action causes such an explosive reaction. If the biting continues, try not to pull away, as you may do yourself more damage. Instead, hold him into you, so his nose is blocked by your breast. He'll soon let go, so he can breathe freely.

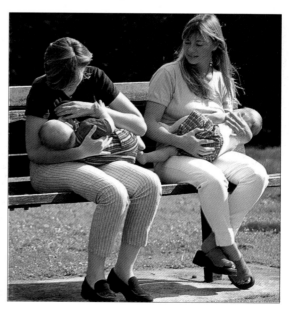

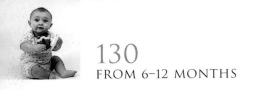

CHILDCARE CHOICES

The most important decision, when you are returning to work, is what kind of childcare you'll need. When you've made your choice, returning to work can then be something to be enjoyed rather than dreaded.

You can choose from different types of childcare, although you may be limited by local availability and your budget. Good childcare is not cheap.

TO MAKE AN INFORMED CHOICE:

• Do your homework thoroughly so that you know what's available well in advance.
• Follow your gut feelings in moments of doubt. Do what feels right to you.
• Do as many checks as possible on your choice, following up references yourself wherever you can. Try to get two references.

NANNY

A nanny would be expected to take sole charge of a baby or child in the child's own home. She would also be expected to shop for and prepare the baby's meals, wash her clothes and keep her room clean and tidy and change bed clothes when needed. In short, she would be responsible for all aspects of her care. She may either live in, or come in on a daily basis.

Approximate budget
£80–260 per week for either a live-in or live-out nanny

(These are net figures. Tax and National Insurance are payable on top.)

Advantages
• You don't have to dress, feed, change the baby or pack up her bag before you leave for work.
• The carer comes to the baby, so there is less disruption for her.
• The nanny becomes part of the family.
• One-to-one care for the baby.
• The other baby chores are done too.

Disadvantages
• It is not necessary for a nanny who comes to the house to be registered with social services.
• Someone else will be in your house all day: your living expenses will rise.
• You are required to become her employer, with attendant responsibilities.

Another alternative is a nanny share, where you and someone else with a baby share the same nanny. This gives companionship for your baby, and halves the costs of your nanny.

CHILDMINDER

A childminder will look after your baby in her own home, which will be registered and regularly inspected by social services. The size of her home puts a restriction on the number of children she can mind.

A childminder is almost always a mother herself. Your child will be cared for with her children and any others that she is minding.

Approximate budget

£50–140 per week

You are likely to be charged at the higher end of the range for babies, as they require more hands-on care.

Advantages

• A childminder is generally an experienced mother.

• Instant group of playmates for baby.

• Home environment.

• Regularly checked by social services.

• Hours can be flexible.

• Registered with social services.

Disadvantages

• Your baby will be more exposed to colds/viruses outside home.

• If childminder is ill, you must make alternative arrangements.

• Some parents worry that childminder will favour their own children.

NURSERY

A nursery may cater for babies and children from the age of three months to five years. Sometimes called a 'crèche' or 'daycare', nurseries are staffed by a combination of qualified nursery nurses and unqualified carers, and there are designated areas and staffing ratios for different age groups. For the under 2s, the staff to baby ratio is 1 to 3. This means nursery care is generally most expensive for the babies.

The nursery will provide care in a stimulating environment with lots of toys and other children. There should be a key worker system in place, whereby all children have one or two carers who are especially responsible for them whom they can get to know well and eventually bond with.

Approximate budget for a private nursery

Up to £30 per day, which tends to be from 7 or 8am until 6.30 or 7pm

Or,

£130 per week

Or, £500 to £600 per month

(These prices vary round the country.)

You may be able to find a state run nursery, but they are few and far between.

If your employer provides a workplace crèche, you should find that this is subsidised.

Advantages

• Stimulating, fun environment, focused on learning through play.

• It will never be closed because of illness.

• Your child will be surrounded by other children.

• It should be registered with social services and therefore is regularly inspected.

Disadvantages

• There are often long waiting-lists.

• Babies are exposed to colds and bugs outside the home.

• The opening hours are not flexible and babies and children have to fit into the nursery routine.

• Some parents think the environment is too busy for babies.

PREPARE FOR THE UNEXPECTED

Prepare a list of emergency helpers to give you back up in case your carer is ill.

If your child is ill, you will need to take time off work. See if your employer provides family leave for such an occurrence. If not, keep a week of your annual leave aside, just in case.

HOW TO FIND YOUR CHILDCARE

Contact your local Social Services department for a list of registered childminders and nurseries.

Contact Nanny agencies and buy newspapers and relevant magazines for nannies, au pairs and mother's helps or advertise locally.

MAKING A CHOICE: IDENTIFYING YOUR NEEDS

In order to make a choice about the best type of childcare for you, it is important to identify your needs, by asking yourself questions about the sort of life you lead, and how you see childcare fitting in. For example:
• Do you want childcare that is home based or do you prefer to drop her off somewhere?
• Do you want a mother-figure to care for your baby?
• Do you want some domestic help too?
• Is it important for your baby to be in a social environment?
• How much can you afford to spend?
• Do you need flexibility in your childcare?

Whichever type of care you prefer, your baby will need:
• a special person or persons with whom she can form an attachment
• consistency of care from the same people
• and carers who will allow her to develop at her own pace.

TWO HEADS ARE BETTER THAN ONE

Your partner should be fully involved in the decision-making process, and meet any prospective carers with you. You should agree to an absolute veto if one of you doesn't like someone. For your child's benefit and future security, all the adults in a child's life should get on well together, because there's no doubt that even if you think they don't know that your nanny or childminder grates on you or your partner, they will learn quickly and play one off against the other.

In the day nursery, look out for:
• a current certificate of registration
• a friendly, drop-in policy for parents
• plenty of evidence of productive play, such as children's pictures on the walls
• a flexible approach to your baby's routine
• a 'key worker' system
• evidence of staff with high morale, such as a low turnover and happy and motivated workers.

INTERVIEWING CHILDMINDERS AND NANNIES

1) In your home

This may be the first time that you have done any interviewing, and you may feel as nervous about the idea as your prospective carer! But with a little time preparing yourself, and a few deep breaths, you will sail through. If you are interviewing in your home, try to get someone to look after the baby for half an hour, so that you can really listen to your interviewee, and build up a picture of her. You should make a list of what you want to discuss, which would probably include the following:
• previous experience
• qualifications
• family background
• attitudes to discipline
• feeding your child
• a job description: what you would expect her to do
• conditions: salary, holidays and notice
• references.

You should give her a chance to ask you questions. Listen carefully to her answers, and, more importantly to what she doesn't say. A strong candidate would be more likely to start by asking you about the child rather than the pay and conditions of the job.

Whilst it is good to have time alone, it is also very important that you see the carer interacting with your baby. Look out for the way they respond to each other.

2) In their home

As well as asking the questions above, have a good look around. Are there toys around for the children to play with? Nobody expects a childminder's house to be spotless, but you would hope that there is nothing that could make a child ill, such as food lying on the floor or small toys lying where a baby could pick them up and swallow them.

You would also need to know about pets, members of the family and how many other children she minds.

MAKING YOUR CHOICE

This may not be easy, but you should always ensure that references are impeccable and even then, if you feel uncomfortable, trust your instinct and be cautious until you are completely satisfied.

Once you have made a choice, you should draw up a contract or agreement between you so that any disagreements in the future can be easily resolved. Many childminders have standard contracts that you can use. Otherwise, it is a good idea for both of you to draw up the contract together.

The contract should cover at least the following: duties, responsibilities, hours, pay, perks (such as use of car, telephone), sick pay, how to plan holidays, length of notice on either side, reasons for termination of contract.

And both of you should sign the contract.

PREPARING FOR CHILDCARE

As the time to return to work grows imminent, prepare for the change so that it is gradual and as seamless an alteration as possible.

If possible, build up the time your baby spends at the childminder. You could spend one or two visits together, leaving for a while on the second visit, so she starts getting used to you being away. If you are returning to work full-time, it would help to start with a week part-time.

ON THE DAY – YOU

If you are taking your baby to a childminder or nursery, you'll need to send a bag with her nappies and change of clothes inside (plus her usual milk and anything else they may tell you to bring). Prepare it the night before.

Do a dummy run the day before, at the time that you would normally do it – see how long it takes in normal conditions.

Leave a list of contact numbers for your carers, which include your number (and extension), your partner's, the GP's, and a relative or friend.

Pack all your gear if you will be expressing milk at work.

Try to schedule any important meetings later in the day.

Ask your carer if they will ring you after a couple of hours, to reassure you all is well.

– YOUR BABY

Make sure she has lots of familiar objects with her: toys, cuddlies, dummies, etc.

Keep as many other things in her life unchanged as possible for the moment. Put your social life on the back burner.

Give plenty of cuddles when you're together.

YOUR BABY FROM 1 YEAR–18 MONTHS

You've made it through the first year! Bake a cake to celebrate your success as parents as well as one for the first birthday party. The past year has been full of new experiences and you've all come a long way.

One year brings an explosion of activity as your little baby turns into a toddler. Having been practising for months, your 12-month-old is now well on the way to walking and talking. All that rolling and crawling will allow her, if she hasn't done it already, to learn to walk alone. She has been communicating since she was born, but now she'll begin to vocalise with great expression and eventually to talk.

She can finally bring together a myriad of physical skills – walking, reaching, grasping, turning – so that suddenly she's an explorer. And each time anything changes, she can explore those changes with renewed vigour. It's almost as though she's seeing those old toys for the first time – realising their potential. But exploring at this age can be a painful business. Your baby's memory is still short and she may stand up under the table and bump herself often before she remembers to crawl out.

Between one year and 18 months, your baby will gradually come to a clearer understanding of how separate you and she really are. It's a long process because you (rightly) try to meet her needs and thereby bolster the illusion that the two of you are inseparable. So this emerging understanding can be a scary business.

NEW RELATIONSHIPS

But little by little your baby is beginning to look out from the intense relationship that you and she have had, to the outer world of brothers and sisters, grandparents, and other children. These secondary relationships will be slow to develop and she will still need you the most.

Between one year and 18 months, the relationship you began with your baby at birth becomes clearer. Understanding how babies learn to relate to other people and how you can help or hinder this process is perhaps one of the

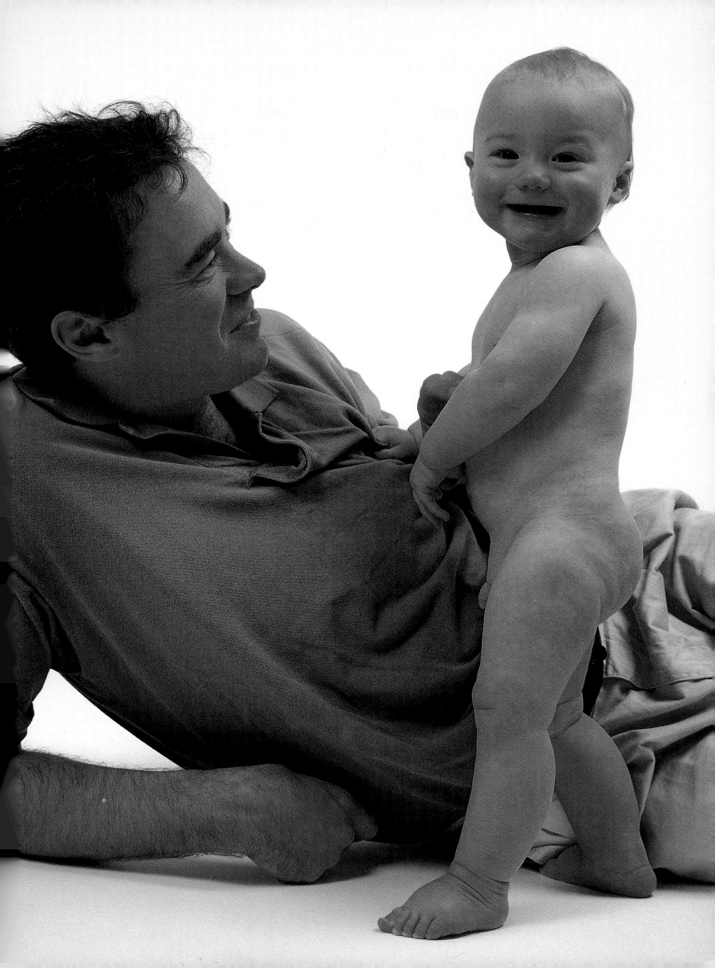

most significant tasks of parenthood. Babies learn what to feel about themselves firstly (usually) from their mums, and secondly (often) from their dads. But they can't learn different lessons from the ones that you live by.

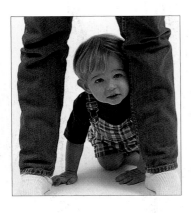

If you love yourself, the chances are your baby will learn to feel good about herself too, and to go through life ensuring that people treat her well. If there are aspects of yourself that you can't accept, then she's likely to feel the same way about herself. Whatever you don't like about yourself – shyness, anger, isolation, loudness, busyness – whatever – talk through your feelings with someone you trust until you are happy to be a model for your baby.

FEELING SECURE

Secure relationships tend to be those in which the parents have consistently responded to their baby's needs, so that the baby feels appreciated, important and loved. Psychologists call this first relationship, an attachment, by which they mean a long-lasting bond between two people – the baby and (usually) the mum.

Attachment has little to do with the amount of time you spend with your baby, and even less with the number of toys you buy her, but has everything to do with tuning in to what she needs. Some babies need a lot of time to themselves, others crave company, some like a lot of action, others to sit quietly and cuddle, and most need a bit of each, at least some of the time. Give her the time that she really needs and she'll be more securely attached to you. To learn that the world is a safe place and that food, comfort and reassurance are on hand when needed, is a vital lesson.

'I have a childminder, one day a week, who takes two of the children, so that I can spend time alone with the third. It's just brilliant.' (Beany, mother of twins pictured here, Oliver and Rebecca, 12 months, and Kim, 3)

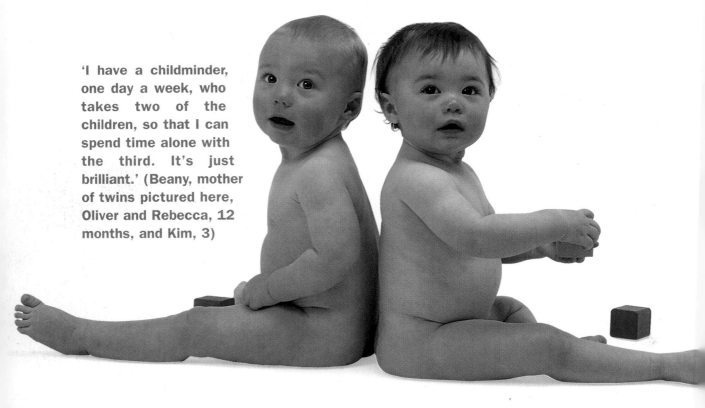

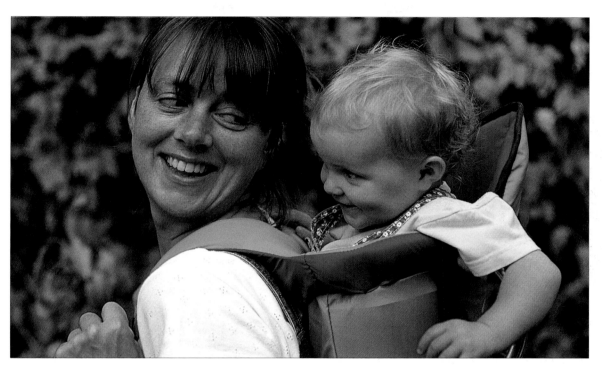

Paradoxically, the more securely attached she is, the more confident she will be to leave you and go off to explore. Once she's full of love and self-worth she can go a long way, just so long as she knows you're there when she needs to go back to you and restock.

It's a pattern that she will carry with her into future relationships. A woman who, as a baby, has been taught how to love herself will search out and find other confident, self-assured people; she'll enjoy relationships that are good for her. It's a pattern that, once set, can happily last a life-time.

'The highlight of my day is getting in from work and being jumped on by all the kids!' (Peter, Beany's partner)

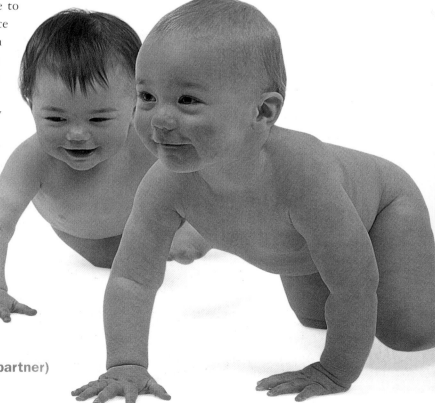

DIARY OF A ONE-YEAR-OLD

Daniel is one year old. His mother, Robin, doesn't work outside the home – looking after Daniel is her full-time job. His father, Chris, works away from home, often for long hours.

5.45am

Chris gets up, which usually wakes Daniel. Robin takes Daniel into bed with her and plays with him, or takes him downstairs and makes a cup of tea while Daniel has a drink and maybe a banana. Daniel is no longer breastfed, having given breastfeeding up of his own accord at seven months.

7am

Daniel likes to watch Teletubbies on the television. He loves the bright colours of the characters and enjoys the fact that he recognises them. He likes playing with balls – 'ba' is one of his two words – so is always delighted to see the Teletubbies' ball.

7.30am

Breakfast, which is usually cereal and some fruit, and sometimes toast. Daniel likes to feed himself, although when he does he tends to wave the spoon full of food around so that it goes everywhere, and to tip the bowl upside down. Robin's compromise is to put the food on the spoon herself then give it to Daniel to put in his mouth.

After breakfast, Daniel plays for a while. He likes toys that he can bash and make a noise with. He particularly enjoys playing with saucepans and baking trays. He also likes books and can now turn the pages of board books for himself. Usually, though, when he picks up a book it's a cue that he wants Robin to play with him.

8.30am

Daniel has a sleep. Robin uses this time for domestic tasks. She finds that it's not always easy to keep Daniel amused while she's doing jobs around the house if he's awake. 'I need to watch him the whole time. He's into everything and doesn't keep still for a minute. I think he's occupied with something, but moments later he wants to do something else,' she says. Daniel has just started climbing up on the furniture, which means that Robin has to watch him particularly closely in case of falls.

10am

Robin wakes Daniel and they get ready to go out. Their mornings are taken up with either shopping, or going swimming, or to a baby and toddler singing group, or to an NCT coffee morning, or for a walk to the river to look at the ducks and feed them.

12noon

Lunchtime. Daniel used to eat more or less anything he was given, but

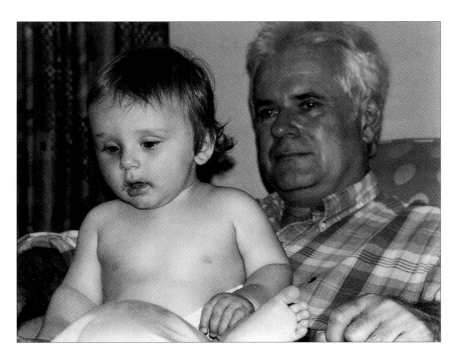

5.30pm
Daniel has his bath. He's recently become interested in toys that pour water and enjoys playing with those in the bath.

6pm
Bedtime. Robin reads to him before he goes to sleep. She enjoys this time because it gives her an opportunity for a cuddle. Daniel isn't generally a cuddly baby – he much prefers being active – but is happy to be cuddled while Robin reads to him.

recently has become faddy about food. 'If he doesn't want it, he throws it on the floor,' Robin says.

1pm
Daniel has another sleep. 'He hurtles round so much that he gets very tired,' says Robin.

2pm
Daniel wakes up and he and Robin either go out again, or go into the garden, or play inside. 'I could easily spend all the time just playing with him,' Robin observes. 'He's very demanding. He hates it if I'm on the phone, for example.' Sometimes she finds herself running out of ideas for ways to keep him entertained. But keeping up with him has some advantages for her: 'I'm losing weight like crazy!'

4.30pm
Robin starts getting Daniel's tea ready. After tea, he plays for a while until it's time to go upstairs for his bath.

Although he protests when Robin leaves him to go to sleep, he usually settles when he realises she's not going back. 'He can be very manipulative,' says Robin. 'We have high drama, but if I go back to him, he laughs. I've now learnt to tell when he's really upset and when he's just screaming to get an audience.'

Robin comments: 'When I put Daniel to bed, I sometimes think, "What have I done today?" and realise that it's been nothing apart from looking after him. But I do have someone who looks after him for a couple of hours twice a week so that I can go to my exercise class and do other things for myself. And I find looking after him very fulfilling. He's such good fun to be with, and I really enjoy watching him change and developing new skills. He's so proud of himself. It's fulfilling too, feeling that I'm doing an important job here, helping him to develop and grow.'

COMMUNICATION AT ONE YEAR

Some babies say their first words at nine months, others not until they are two years old, and boys often talk later than girls. So there's a wide variation.

Between one year and 18 months your baby will be actively listening to what you say and the way that you say it and may be taking his first tentative stabs at a few words. If your child isn't talking at all by the time he's two, take him for a hearing test, it may be that repeated hearing problems are delaying his speech.

First words are likely to be the names of things that are important to your baby and to be shorter than the conventional words: 'ma' and 'da' for 'mummy' and 'daddy'. One sound may mean many things: 'cah' for 'car', 'cat' and 'cup'. But the context usually helps you sort out the 'cup' from the 'car'.

And as he learns the words for the things around him, your baby will continue to use gestures like looking, pointing and waving to communicate.

HOW YOU CAN HELP

What he most needs from you is a lot of one-to-one, positive conversation so that he can frequently hear the sounds he'll eventually produce, and feel motivated to use them.

Times when you could enjoy chatting together are, for example, when you're going round the supermarket together, with him perched in the shopping trolley facing you. He'll probably reach out for items off the shelves and you can supply the word he's looking for, or ask his opinion about what to buy. Most toddlers love the trolley.

AT ONE YEAR

- turns to the sound of his name
- understands many familiar words and instructions
- plays 'pat-a-cake'
- waves 'bye-bye'
- points at things when they interest him.

AT 15 MONTHS

- imperious finger pointing
- speaks two to six recognisable words, understands many more
- asks for what he wants at the table by pointing and vocalising.

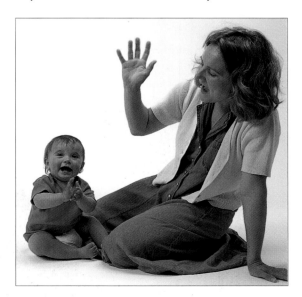

Another good talking opportunity is bedtime. Talking through the events of the day or singing lullabies will stimulate his interest in words: nursery rhymes are particularly good for increasing verbal awareness.

A constant background noise of radio or the TV could interfere with his picking up language, or mean that he can't get your attention enough to succeed at communicating, so switch it off from time to time.

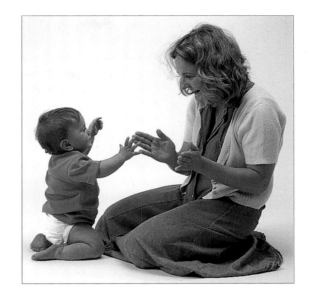

HELP YOUR TODDLER TALK

- have some time without the television or radio on, so that you can chat
- talk to your toddler one-to-one; make it fun
- sing nursery rhymes; read repetitive stories
- talk about what you're doing as you do it, so that your toddler can match the context to the words: 'Here's your mug', 'It's bath time now', 'Which fruit shall we buy?'
- look directly at him when you speak
- make him feel that you value what he has to say, even though it may be hard to understand
- leave him a space to answer if he likes, but don't insist that he does so.

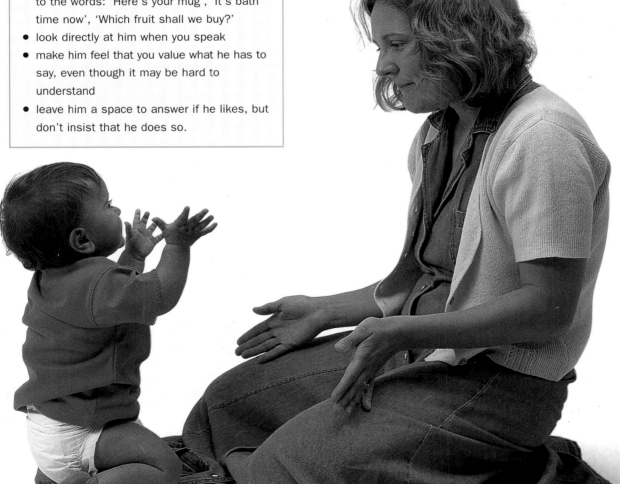

PHYSICAL SKILLS AT ONE YEAR

New skills are developing speedily at 12 months. As well as manipulating toys in new ways, he will find clever new games to play with you.

At one year, your baby will probably know what many things are for but she won't yet have mastered their use. She may 'comb' her hair with the wrong side of the comb, or struggle to scoop some food in her spoon and then tip most of it out again before it reaches her mouth. You'll still need to feed her most of the time if she's not to starve. Most babies fare a little better with their cup, although this too can be messy. 'Elliott (14 months) tends to do his holy water act with his beaker – and sprinkle it about.'

By now your baby will be able to imitate repetitive actions like waving bye-bye, although typically (and frustratingly) just as your visitor turns away. Pat-a-cake is another favourite game at about a year, as she is now able to voluntarily open her hands and co-ordinate bringing them together. But she may have to wait a few years yet until she masters flamenco.

MORE POWER TO HER ARM

By the time she gets to 15 months your toddler may be able to copy a tower of two bricks though she probably still finds it more fun to knock yours down. She's learnt that flat sides balance best, and that squaring up the bricks stops the finished product looking like the Leaning Tower of Pisa. And her arms are sufficiently under her

control to allow her to place the top brick.

But her arms still mostly move in one plane at a time. Give her a crayon and she may hold it in her fist and draw backwards and forwards over some paper if you show her how, but she won't be able to go around in circles or make dots, those complicated arm movements are beyond her.

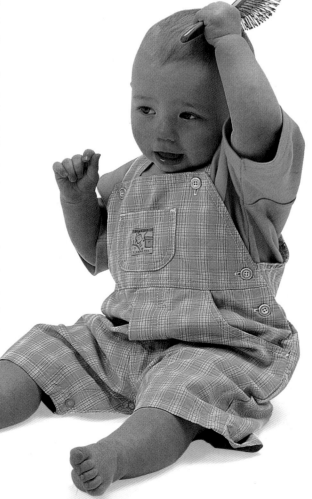

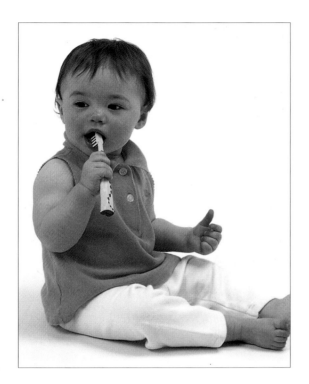

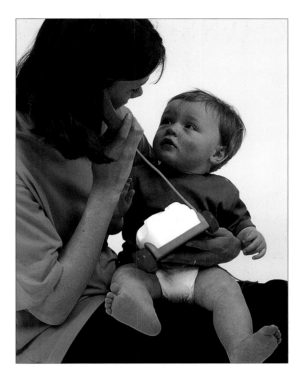

At 15 months your baby will explore toys to see how they can be used, banging, poking, shaking, rolling and pushing them. She'll start to use them as tools if she can. By now she'll seldom put things in her mouth, but will stare intently at things that interest her. The more buttons, dials, sounds and sensations a toy has the more she'll love it. And now that she's mobile, she'll want to get hold of everything that she can get at. Watch out!

HANDEDNESS

When babies first discover their hands they use both equally. By about six months some show a preference for one hand, and many more prefer one over the other by about a year. However, some children remain ambidextrous until they are four, five or six. Even when your baby begins to show a preference for one hand. she will continue to develop her ability with both. For example, by 15 months most babies have developed a pincer grip (thumb and forefinger grip) and pick up small items equally well with either hand.

Most children are right-handed, but there is increasing awareness that being left-handed is neither a handicap nor something that can be changed. If you try to change your baby from using his left to using his right hand you are likely to make him confused and frustrated, but you're unlikely to get him to change his ways. And now there are left-handed pens, scissors and even corkscrews, where's the problem?

Better by far to concentrate on helping your baby to develop control and strength in both hands by sometimes offering him a toy to one hand and sometimes to the other.

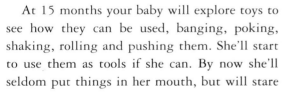

CRUISING AND COASTING

Learning to walk begins with your baby's first attempt to stand. At first, she'll distribute her weight between hands and feet but it won't be long before she's just using hands for balance.

Some time after nine months your baby will begin to pull herself up to standing, but like all her new-found skills she's better at starting than she is at stopping, and the only way back down again is with a bump onto her bottom, or by calling for you. It takes her a few weeks to get the hang of sticking out her bottom. But meanwhile your baby just loves to stand – the view from there is so much better than the view from the floor – so no sooner has she bumped down, or been helped down, than she is pulling herself back up again, on anything from people to furniture to walls: 'Florence (15 months) has this uncanny knack

of climbing up my leg just when I've got to rush somewhere'.

If you hold on to one or both of her hands at this time she will love to step purposefully on alternate feet. And once she's learnt the trick, hey presto! she can cruise or coast around the furniture, side stepping as she goes. You may have to decorate accordingly: 'I've noticed how the contents of my rooms have changed from porcelain to plastic, and from pretty colours to primaries,' says one toddler's mum. Some time after a year your baby may let go of whatever she pulled herself up on and stand on her own, cowboy-style, with feet widely spread for balance.

A push-along toy with wheels and a heavy base will help him get his confidence walking. He will use the handle to pull

Now that Oliver (12 months) can put one foot in front of the other, push-along toys are great fun

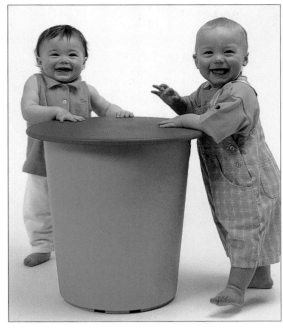

is satisfactory speed of movement with sit-in walkers they are not good for the ankles when used for long periods of time.

Other toys that help to develop the leg muscles are tricycles and ride-ons. If he can sit on a toy truck and propel himself along by pushing against the floor, the next step could be learning to pedal, which takes a considerable amount of co-ordination and is the first step in learning to ride a bike.

himself up to standing, so make sure the toy is strong enough to take this treatment without tipping over. Avoid lightweight wheelbarrows and dolls' buggies which won't take his weight.

Push-along walkers are better than the circular kind of baby-walker where the child sits in the middle of the toy and propels himself along without using the hands. Although there

'Sophie (15 months) seems to have decided that she's ready to walk down the stairs forwards, like the rest of us. I wasn't worried about her on the stairs until now.'

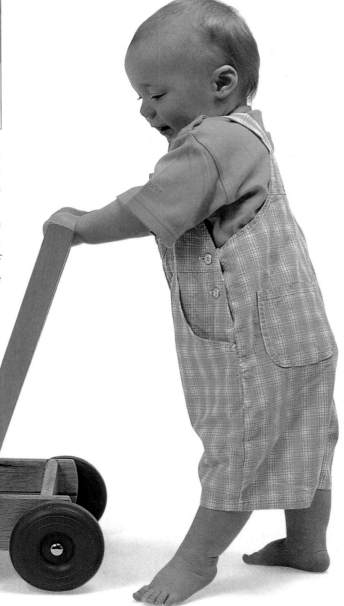

WALKING INDEPENDENTLY

Once he's comfortable balancing all his weight on legs and feet and is able to move confidently as long as he's holding on, the day will come when he'll feel strong enough to let go.

By the time she is 15 months old your baby will probably be able to get to her feet under her own steam, without hoisting herself up on someone or something. The next step will be her first step. The average baby walks on her own, albeit unevenly, at about 14 or 15 months and stops by falling over or bumping into furniture. More a lurch than a walk – but wonderful none the less. It's definitely worth hiring a camcorder at this stage to get it all on video.

A few babies walk as early as nine months

and a few more not until they are two years old. Such variation is quite normal, but if your baby isn't walking by 18 months and you are worried, ask your doctor to check her over.

Games that you can play with your baby, to encourage walking, include placing low-level furniture carefully around the room so that she can move from one support to the next without crawling. Move the items of furniture an inch or two apart as her confidence increases.

You could also try crouching down in front of her and holding out your arms for her to stagger into. You will probably find that you do this

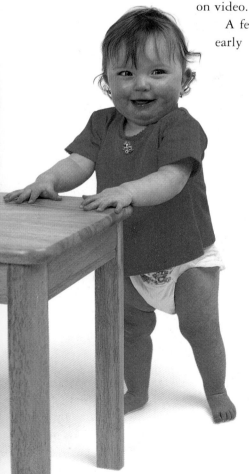

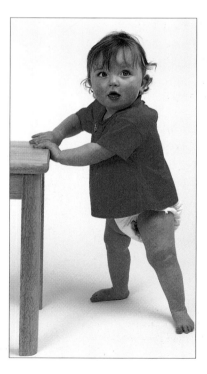

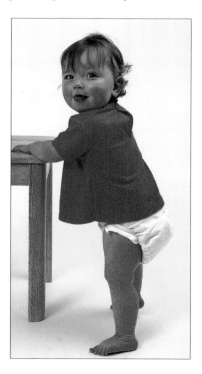

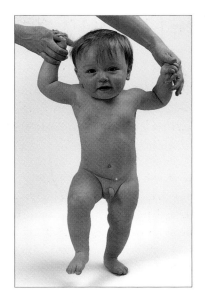

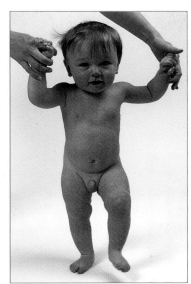

STANDING ALONE

To stand alone your baby needs four things: to be able to stretch out his hips and his knees, to have strong leg muscles, and to be able to balance. If any of these is missing he will stand later. However, if your baby isn't standing by 16 months make an appointment to have a chat with your doctor.

naturally, without even thinking about it, as you see her attempting to let go of supporting furniture and step free. Gradually increase the distance so that she has slightly further to stagger towards you each time (without upsetting her, obviously). Give her lots of cuddles and encouragement as she achieves each milestone on the way to real walking. The more practice your baby has, the sooner she'll develop her co-ordination and learn to do it.

Shoes are not needed at this stage. It's actually easier for her to keep her balance if she can feel the floor beneath the soles of her feet and can use her toes to stay upright. Shoes are only needed for a lot of walking along pavements, and they will feel very odd on her feet at first. Socks may be all that's needed to keep her feet warm, but will be dangerously slippery on polished floors.

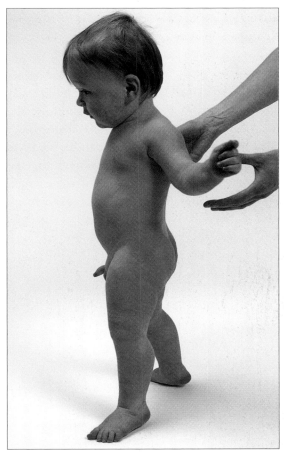

Although Max and Amelia are year-old twins, Max (above) is more advanced than his sister at learning to walk and is nearly there. Amelia (see left) is at the earlier stage and still side-stepping around the furniture

FEEDING AND SELF-FEEDING

As your baby grows and becomes accustomed to solid food, you will be able to offer him a good variety. Even if he doesn't enjoy all the tastes, he will benefit from the array of choices now available to him.

By around a year, the number of different foods that your baby can enjoy will gradually increase. This means a mixed diet that will include a number of dairy foods, such as fromage frais, yoghurt and cheese (still not soft or blue cheeses, though), proteins such as beans, chicken, white fish and lamb, cereals such as bread, pasta, breakfast cereals and rice, and finally, fruit and vegetables.

'She'll try a new taste in the morning and loves it, but then won't eat it in the evening.'

As the variety widens, so the texture of the foods can gradually become more challenging. When he first started on solids, all his food was probably very smooth and runny. Now you can make it lumpier, so he learns to chew more. Food will become more interesting, as there are now different colours, shapes, and textures as well as tastes.

GROWING INDEPENDENCE

Food is a colourful and sensual adventure and of course, he will want to touch it, squeeze it through his fingers, push it in his hair, and perhaps get some in his mouth. This is an important developmental stage which he will thoroughly enjoy, even if you don't.

Accept this as a learning stage and prepare your kitchen and his clothes for the onslaught:

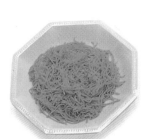

• Place a large plastic mat under his high chair that should catch most of the food that heads for the floor.
• Offer him a plastic spoon/s of his own so he can try to feed himself.
• Keep spare bibs handy.
• Remove any 'good' clothes (particularly if he is eating banana, which never comes out).
• Use a bowl with a suction pad on the bottom.

FINGER FOODS

One way that your baby can learn to feed himself is by offering plenty of finger foods. This both encourages him to eat independently, and develops his fine motor skills. Take care with hard foods, such as raw carrot or celery, as he may now bite off large pieces which he can't chew up and start to choke. Foods that can be

THE RIGHT DIET FOR BABIES

Your baby will need plenty of energy-giving foods to help him grow and develop to his full potential. Whilst adults are encouraged to follow a healthy diet which is high in fibre and low in fat, this is not the ideal combination for babies. Too much fibre is difficult to digest and babies need plenty of fat for growth.

sucked into a pulp are best at first, such as fingers of toast, or bread sticks, or small, soft items such as cooked pasta or pieces of grated cheese. Never leave your baby alone while he is eating, in case of choking.

Some
other finger foods are:
•slices of melon •kiwi fruit
•apple •pear •peach •banana •grated
carrot •grated apple •strawberry •avocado
•rice cakes •little sandwiches •pieces of
cooked vegetables •cucumber •bits of chicken

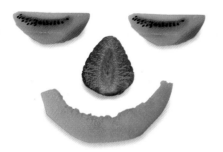

DRINKS

Milk will still be an important part of your baby's diet. Although he can have small quantities of cow's milk mixed with cereals or porridge once he is six months old, his milk feeds should be either breast milk or formula milk until he is a year old. If you want to give him any other fluids, you can offer him some cooled, boiled water. There is a tempting array of fruit juices available for young babies.

> You should still be avoiding the following:
> Salt/Sugar/Highly spiced or cured meats
> High fibre foods
> Fizzy or sugary drinks
> Whole or chopped nuts

If you give these to your young baby, you may encourage a liking for sweetened drinks that may be hard to cure in the future. If you do offer fruit juice, mix it with water.

PART OF THE FAMILY

By the middle of the second year, your baby will be able to take his place at the family meal. He should find meal-times happy occasions, a social event where the family members meet, at least some of the time. He will enjoy taking his place more if meal times are unhurried and

> **'It's important, as he gets older, for him to feel that he can do it himself.'**

he can do as much as possible by himself. By now you should know what he enjoys and can offer him favourites together with a new taste every so often.

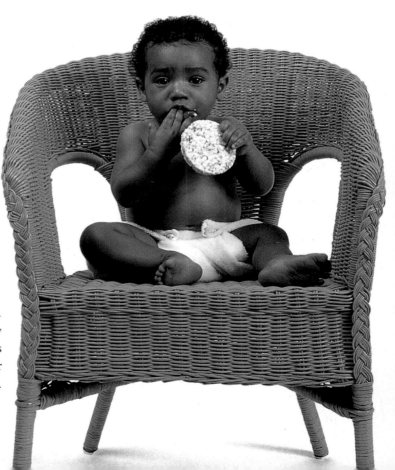

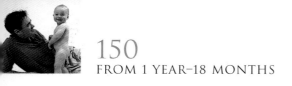

SEPARATION ANXIETY

Although it can be a nuisance to have your every visit to the loo accompanied, separation anxiety is normal and a good indication that your baby is developing a close relationship with you.

You know your baby is suffering from separation anxiety when he doesn't like you to go out of his sight. His model of the world is based on the idea that even if the two of you are not one and the same, at least the natural state of affairs is togetherness, so when you try to leave him alone, he's frightened.

The most helpful thing you can do is go with it. The fact that he's clingy now doesn't mean he'll be clingy forever. In fact, he's likely to get over the clinging stage of dependency more quickly if you let him have as much of you as he wants right now. Once he understands that even when you disappear you soon come back, he'll re-find his confidence.

'We get to the crèche at about 8am and so long as I sit him down to breakfast, Callum (17 months) is happy to let me go.'

Some psychologists believe that the way a one-year-old acts when his mother leaves him in an unfamiliar place is a good indication of the quality of the relationship. Babies who cling to their mother, even when she stays with them in a strange place, may be demonstrating that they cannot rely on their mother to always be there, so they dare not let her go. Similarly, babies who show no upset when their mother leaves them, may not have formed a close enough relationship with her. On the other hand, a baby who protests when his mother leaves, but welcomes her back with smiles and hugs is, it is claimed, securely attached.

At round about a year, your baby may develop a liking for particular toys or objects. This is part of her increasing awareness of the differences between things, and an expression of her emerging personality. Some of these toys may become more than just favourite playthings; your baby may feel that she cannot get through difficult situations without them. Babies start to use these toys for cuddling, rather than playing and often cuddle in the same way each time – holding their cuddly while twiddling their hair, or sucking their thumb or stroking their cheek, for example. Psychologists call these comforters 'transitional objects'. 'Transitional' because your baby uses her teddy, or a piece of your old dressing gown, as a substitute for you.

CUDDLIES

Transitional objects come in many shapes and sizes, from bottles and dummies to old blankets and even silky underwear. It's estimated that around 70% of children have a 'cuddly' of some description. What characterises them is the importance that they have in babies' lives.

Children who are struggling with separation anxiety get very worried about losing mum (or whoever their primary carer might be). They're also beginning to move off on their own, literally learning to walk, and this means all sorts of new possibilities of independence which are really quite scary. A clever solution to this dilemma is to find something to hold on to that can represent security: something that she can take with her whenever she's parted from you.

If the comfort object is a rag, it will probably have a particular texture – either rough or silky – that the baby finds consoling to suck or rub near the mouth. This probably recreates the sensation, when she was breast or bottle-feeding, of having your silky blouse or jumper pressed against her cheek. The texture, smell and even temperature of the cloth can become very important. Wise parents will cut the cloth in half and keep the spare piece in a safe place as an emergency replacement for whenever the first one gets lost.

THUMB-SUCKING

A thumb can also be a comfort object, of course. The area just behind the upper gums in a baby's mouth is very sensitive and sucking is the most basic comfort habit of all. Your baby may suck fingers, thumb or a dummy and refine on the pleasure by fiddling with an earlobe or twisting her hair. Sucking on a thumb has an advantage over sucking on a dummy, in that the thumb cannot get lost. On the other hand, it may be easier for parents to 'lose' the dummy if they want to discourage the habit.

On the whole, the need for a comfort object diminishes when your toddler gets to three or four years old – although thumbs and teddies may still be called upon at times of stress in later life.

But there's no evidence either way that comfort objects help or hinder babies' later development. Probably the best idea is to accept your baby's decision, whatever it is.

YOUR BABY FROM 18 MONTHS–2 YEARS

Sometime between 18 months and two years, your toddler will grasp the powerful idea that one thing can represent another. This understanding is what fuels the sudden leap forward in his development.

Your toddler is ready to leave helpless babyhood behind. He's now beginning to take control of what happens to him. Most of the time, he's still at the mercy of whatever the day brings, but he now begins to think (just a little) about what he will do before he does it.

SEEING THE FUNNY SIDE

This new understanding that one thing can represent another explains the first jokes. Things often seem funny when we expect one thing to happen – but something else does instead. So long as the unexpected isn't frightening, it can be funny. Now that your toddler has a clearer idea of what to expect in many situations, he may be ready to be amused. Put a bowl on your head instead of a hat, or offer him a spade instead of a spoon to eat his food and he may laugh. (If he looks confused or cries,

that's because he's not ready for a joke yet, so leave it a few months.)

From his earliest days, your baby will have been able to imitate you. At first it was facial expressions, then the sound of your voice, movements of parts of his body, and now whole actions. At 18 months, your toddler will love to follow you around and imitate chores as you do them. He'll also still be imitating in other ways. 'Elliott (15 months) saw a nodding cockerel in a shop window and stood outside nodding his head up and down and laughing.'

His ability to imitate will be enhanced by his understanding that one thing can represent another. Once he sees that a towel wrapped around teddy can 'be a baby', he can imitate his mum feeding his little brother. And once he sees that wearing daddy's shoes 'turns him into' daddy he can do a better impression altogether.

It's really no surprise that toddlers recognise themselves in mirrors or photographs for the

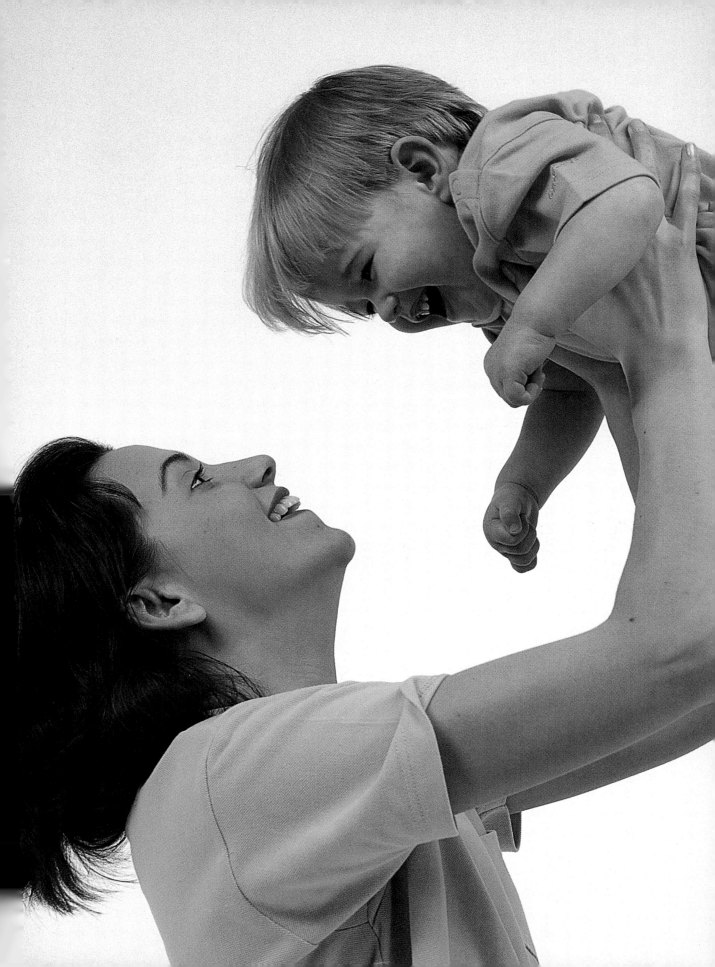

first time at round about this age. Photographs and reflections are both ways in which we can represent ourselves. Your toddler has learnt that his reflection represents himself. But more than just having an idea of his appearance, your toddler is also beginning to have a sense of himself as an individual. If he can see himself in the mirror then there must be a self there to be seen. And this self does things as well as looks a certain way. Your toddler may spend a long time gazing at himself, making faces and moving parts of his body in view of the mirror, experimenting with the idea that he can make all this happen. Most toddlers can recognise themselves by the time they are 21 months. Before this time a baby will gaze at his reflection, or photograph as though he were looking at another baby – he may even look behind the mirror to see where the other baby is.

LANGUAGE

Another way in which your toddler now demonstrates that he understands that one thing can represent another, is by using words. The first words that toddlers learn are those for the important things around them – words like

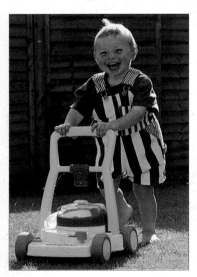

'mummy', 'daddy', 'Tom' and 'Katy' which represent significant people, and other words like 'dink' (for drink), 'bic' (for biscuit) and 'bath' which represent important things.

Initially he may overextend the use of some words. For example, 'As soon as we got here (on

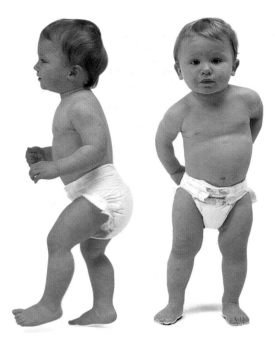

holiday) we drove down to the beach. Hannah (22 months) stood for a long time looking out at the sea and finally said "bath"'.

And 'Isabel (15 months) has just started saying "Daddy", but I find it really embarrassing when she calls every man we meet for the first time "Daddy". People will talk!'.

This labelling process speeds up intellectual development. It will help your toddler learn more quickly by giving him useful pegs on which to hang anything new that he discovers. Language helps your toddler to sort things out.

EXPERIMENTING

Now that your toddler can think (just a little), before he acts he is ready to move on from exploring what's around him to experimenting with it. Those toys that he's been picking up and squishing, throwing, chewing and banging are now more carefully and deliberately, picked up, squished, thrown, chewed and banged. He's beginning to bring his mind and not just his fingers and mouth to bear on the things he finds around him. Your toddler wants to understand.

will have difficulty remembering what groups he is sorting things into. So that faced with a box of different kinds of toys, he might initially begin to pick out all the cars and then half way through, prompted by a spate of yellow cars, change to picking out all the yellow things. What things do and how things look vie for his attention. And with only the beginnings of mental concepts to help him, he is constantly at the mercy of what he sees in front of him.

You could help him by suggesting different categories for him to find – like all the dolls or trains or bricks in a toy box – and sitting with him while he finds them.

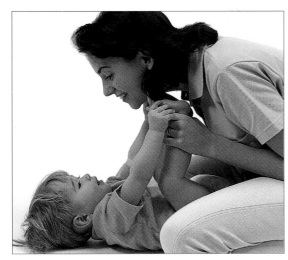

For the first time he acts deliberately and then watches to see what happens. He pats a ball and it rolls a little way along the ground in a straight line, he pats a brick and it turns once and sits still. He couldn't tell you why it is that things with flat sides don't roll, but he's noticed the difference.

Once he has understood about similarities and differences, your toddler is ready to begin to sort things into groups. The trouble is, that everything fits into more than one group and initially at least he

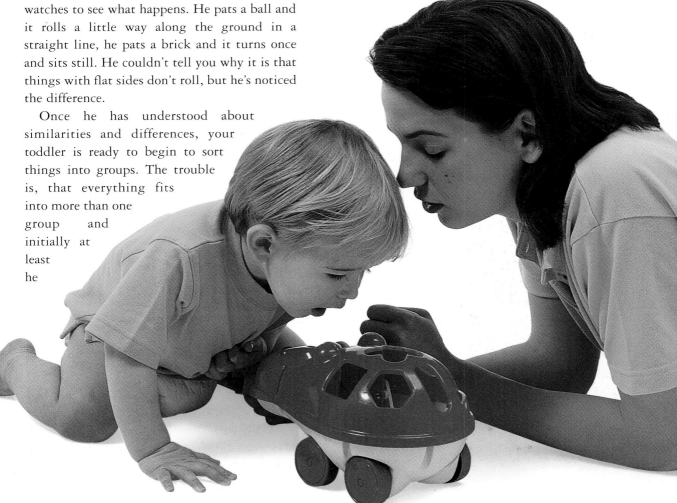

DIARY OF AN 18-MONTH-OLD

Joseph is 18 months old. He goes to a childminder two mornings a week, while his mother, Alice, works. His father, Dave, is out at work during the day.

7am

Joseph wakes up and gets himself out of bed. He's been sleeping in a bed for the last month. If his nappy is only wet, he'll play on his own in his room, talking to his cuddly toys. Alice is by now half-awake and lies in bed listening to him play. If his nappy is dirty, he lets Alice or Dave know that it needs changing.

Nappy-changing has to be done with Joseph standing up as he objects strongly to lying down and won't stay still.

7.30am

Joseph, Alice and Dave have breakfast together. Joseph sits in his highchair and feeds himself his cereal and toast.

After breakfast, Joseph plays by himself while Dave gets ready for work and Alice, if she's not working that day, clears away the breakfast things.

8am

Dave leaves for work. Joseph stands at the door with Alice and waves goodbye to Dave. He likes Alice always to say the same thing – 'Daddy's going to work in his car now'. 'The ritual is important to him,' says Alice.

During the morning, Joseph and Alice play. Sometimes Joseph has a low point around 9.30am, when, as Alice says, 'you can see his alertness plummet.' If this happens, she either puts him to bed to sleep for an hour, or they sit quietly and read books. He especially likes books that have clear pictures of things that he can point to and name. His vocabulary is growing by the day.

Joseph's favourite play activity is making things with Duplo, particularly aeroplanes. He also enjoys playing with Duplo animals, and has just started to play pretend games with them, pretending to feed them. Another favourite game is putting lids on plastic storage containers, though he can't always manage this and gets frustrated with it. If the weather's fine, Joseph and Alice may go out and play in the garden, often in the sandpit. Joseph usually needs a bath after this.

11.30am

If Joseph hasn't had a sleep earlier in the morning, he has a nap for about an hour. Alice gets on with whatever housework needs doing.

12.30pm

Lunchtime. Joseph has a cooked lunch, which he can mostly eat by himself, though he occasionally needs help

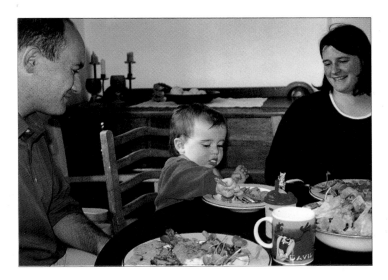

with things that don't stay on the fork very well. Following a recent visit to an admirable three-year-old cousin who willingly ate such things as carrots and broccoli, Joseph will now eat more or less anything.

2pm

Joseph and Alice go out, either to the park, or to visit friends with children the same age as Joseph, or to a toddler group. Joseph makes it quite clear when he wants to go out, picking up his shoes and taking them to Alice, saying 'shoe'. Alternatively, he starts telling Alice the names of the people he'd like to go and see. 'He has a real desire to be with other kids and other adults,' says Alice, 'I'm not enough for him all the time any more.'

4.30pm

Joseph and Alice come home and have a snack. Joseph is often tired and cross by this time. 'Me too,' says Alice. They sit quietly, with Joseph on Alice's lap, often with his dummy, reading books. If Joseph is very overtired and wound-up, as he can be if he's had a demanding afternoon, Alice sometimes gives him a bath to calm him down.

5.30pm

Dave comes home. Alice cooks dinner, while Dave plays games with Joseph.

6pm

Joseph, Alice and Dave have dinner together. After dinner, Dave plays with Joseph again. 'He gets down on the floor with Joseph and gets really involved with him,' comments Alice. 'I sometimes wonder who's the bigger kid. But I love to watch them together.' Joseph especially likes to play hiding games with Dave, standing behind the curtain and calling ''iding'.

6.45pm

Time for bed. Alice will have said to Joseph several times while he was playing with Dave that it's nearly bedtime, so he's prepared for it. He usually goes up to bed quite willingly. After he's had his teeth brushed, he gets into bed with his teddies and Alice says goodnight to him. They always play an intimate little game of touching faces. Once she's said goodnight three or four times, she leaves the room and closes the door. Sometimes Joseph protests at her going, but as Alice says, 'you've got to be firm'. She listens outside the door to make sure he's not really distressed and, on the whole, the protest soon dies down. Once he's gone to sleep, Joseph usually doesn't wake till morning.

Alice comments: 'Joseph's not so much a baby now – more a little child. I actually found the baby bit quite hard, but this is much more rewarding. I love the way he's learning new words all the time, and learning to do new things. And I really enjoy his companionship – he's like a little friend.'

COMMUNICATION AT 18 MONTHS

From now until she is about six years old, your toddler will learn words at the astonishing rate of six to ten new ones every day. It's when talking takes off.

Your 18-month-old toddler will probably jabber loudly and continuously while she plays. She may only have six to 20 words but she will use them often and to mean a wide range of things. Sometimes she will only have to hear words once to remember them especially if you stress them. So if you stub your toe – remember to count to ten before you say anything!

At the same time toddlers learn to combine two words – usually

an 'action' word (not always a verb) and an 'object' word as in 'Mummy come', 'Jack drink'. However, right now your baby's most useful two words will probably be 'what that?' as she strives to name more and more of the things which are important to her. Other favourites are 'more' as in 'more biscuit' or 'more story' and 'again' or 'another'. There's also 'all-gone' pronounced as if it is one word, as in 'all-gone daddy'.

This is the time to get out the saucepan lids and wooden spoons and strike up the kitchen band because at 18 months your toddler will love to join in with nursery rhymes and songs, even if she sings the same line over and over again, and all spectacularly out of tune. Try singing a couple of rounds of 'Heads and shoulders, knees and toes (knees and

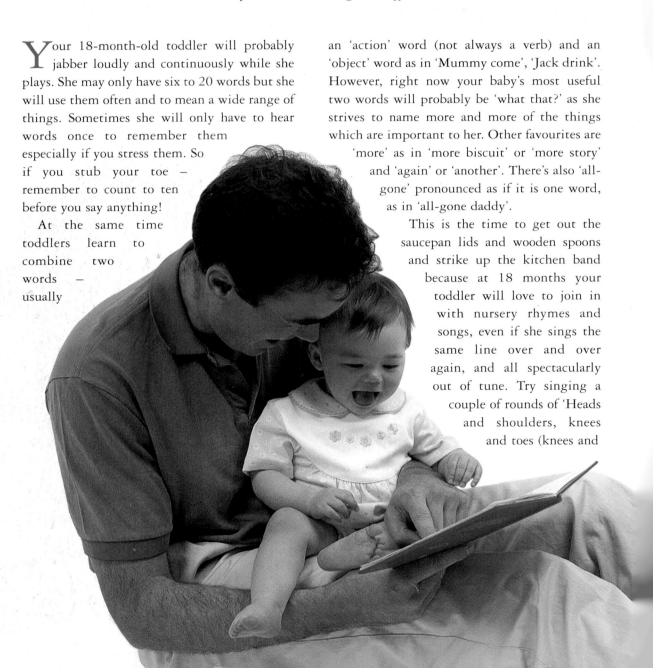

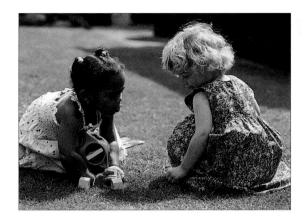

toes)' with her and ask her to point to the appropriate parts of the body with you. You may be surprised at how quickly she learns the right names.

LOOKS AND GLANCES

But toddlers are not just learning what to say they are also practising how to say it. At 18 months your toddler will use the same looks and glances as you do in conversation. She will look at you when you talk and then look away again as if waiting to reply and then glance back, ready to have her turn. When she is talking, your toddler will tend to look at you until she is ready to stop talking and then glance away again, looking back to give you the chance to reply.

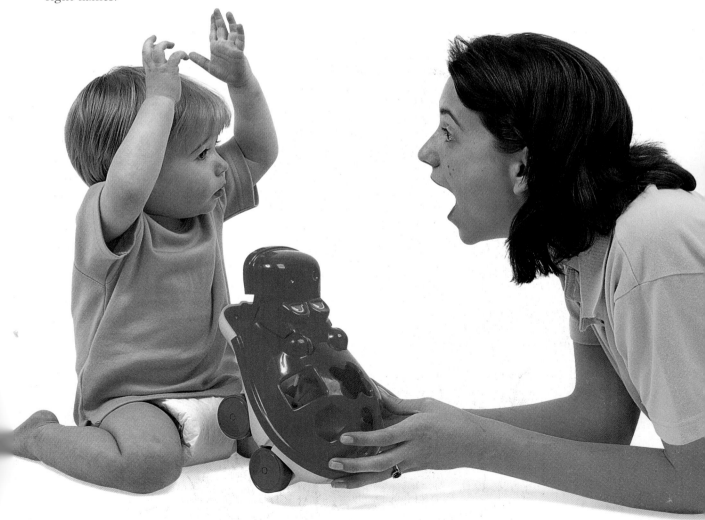

PLAY AT 18 MONTHS

As his walking becomes steadier, your toddler's play moves into a bigger dimension. Mobile babies begin to gain access to a whole new range of experiences.

At 18 months your toddler may have a special toy, it's almost always large and the unfortunate thing has to go everywhere he goes. You'll also find it sharing his meals at mealtimes, if not his bed at night.

As he becomes more confident at walking, large toys with wheels that he can push or pull come into their own. He may like a doll's pushchair or a nodding dog on a string. So long as it keeps its balance, is heavy enough to resist uncontrolled tugs and looks or sounds interesting, it will be a favourite. The fact that many push-along or pull-along toys can also be used in imaginative play, means that they will become increasingly popular and will last your toddler for longer.

'Richard (20 months) has a set of toy kitchen utensils that he carries with him. He's always dropping one and then struggling to pick it up without losing the others.'

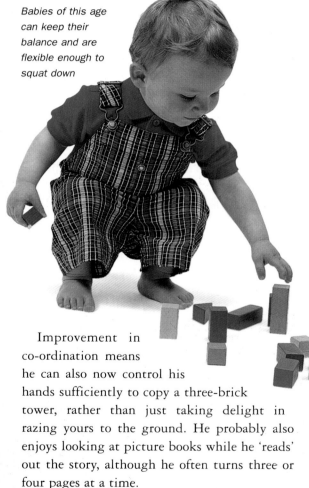

Babies of this age can keep their balance and are flexible enough to squat down

Improvement in co-ordination means he can also now control his hands sufficiently to copy a three-brick tower, rather than just taking delight in razing yours to the ground. He probably also enjoys looking at picture books while he 'reads' out the story, although he often turns three or four pages at a time.

Generally, he'll be happy playing alone or near to other toddlers so long as you are in sight, but he will want to chop and change what he's doing every minute or so, so you'll need to be imaginative in your choice of toys.

At 18 months a simple climbing frame will

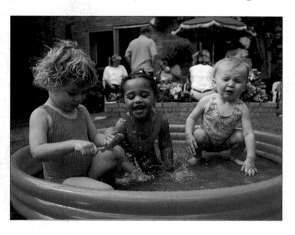

FUN TOYS FOR EXPERIMENTS

Sand, water and playdough are all great for scientific investigations during the second year. They are also amazing fun. Water can be poured and splashed, sand can be trickled when dry, or built with when wet, and playdough (as long as he doesn't instantly put it into his mouth) can be squished, pulled, patted, and endlessly reshaped. (See page 197.)

There's a lot for your toddler to discover when he has access to these three and just one or two simple props like a container for filling and pouring or a blunt knife for cutting. What he will need from you is a quick demonstration of all the different things he could do, the chance to make his own progress, and your help when things don't go as expected.

be popular, if you can find one with a few steps up and a slide down. After they have learned to walk, children also enjoy crawling through tunnels. There is something about being enclosed in a small space that toddlers love. You can either buy a play tunnel from a toyshop or just throw sheets or a tablecloth over a washing line in the garden – or table in the front room – to make a cosy little house or den.

Not many adults could achieve the balance and flexibilty that Luke shows

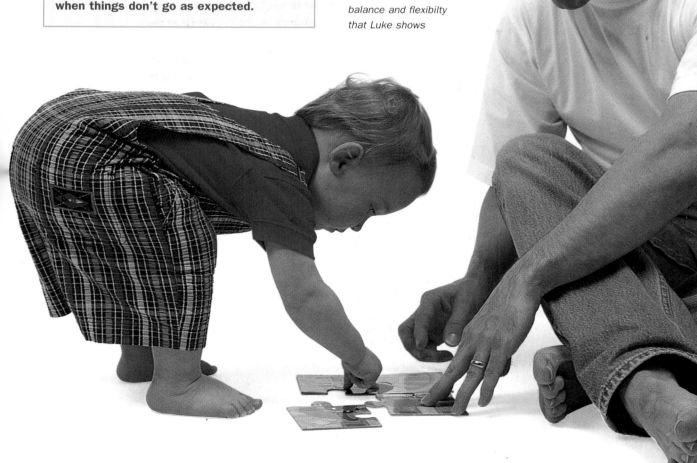
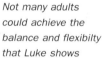

PHYSICAL SKILLS AT 18 MONTHS

By 18 months your toddler's balance will have improved, making a whole lot of new physical skills possible.

Now that she doesn't have to concentrate so hard on her walking, your toddler can begin to build on that skill. She will also have learnt how to stop and start without falling over, whereas a few months ago standing still would have required a massive effort of concentration which frankly wasn't worth it. This new walking ability allows her time to make a decision about where to go next, rather than lumbering haphazardly from one piece of furniture to the next. However, her balance is still not perfect and turning a corner still involves travelling in a semi-circle with arms raised high for balance. Another skill she's probably learnt is the ability to squat. This is invaluable when she makes a find (a snail, a leaf or a drain) but wants to be able to move swiftly on as soon as she's bored.

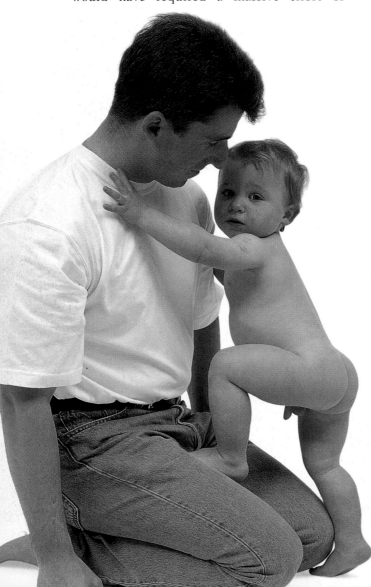

She may even be able to run in a straight line too. But here she reaches the limit of her balancing act – she can negotiate around objects while she's walking, but at full pelt, anything in her way means a crash.

But perhaps the most exciting and potentially dangerous new skill is her ability to climb on and off furniture. Some toddlers seem to climb almost as soon as they can walk whereas other, perhaps more considerate souls, leave that challenge for another few months yet. Climbers will have to be watched with vigilance to make sure that they don't get hurt while exploring.

Physical skills like walking and running, improve with practice. Here's how you can help:

• Give your toddler lots of opportunity to practise.

• Encourage her to be as active as possible.

• Accept that her skills will develop slowly – where practice is concerned, a little and often is better than all or nothing.

• Help her to feel competent and positive about her abilities.

• If one activity is frustrating lead her to another she can do well. She'll want to get it right. Don't push her harder than she pushes herself.

• Make it fun.

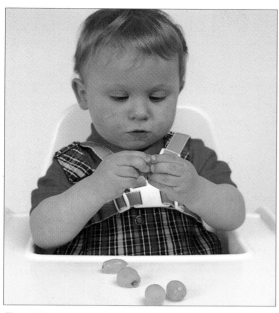

Finger foods are good news for toddlers now and do help to improve their hand–eye co-ordination

'Joseph (18 months) is fascinated by the ants in the garden. Yesterday he poked his finger in the ant hole, and then poked the cracks in the patio with a stick.'

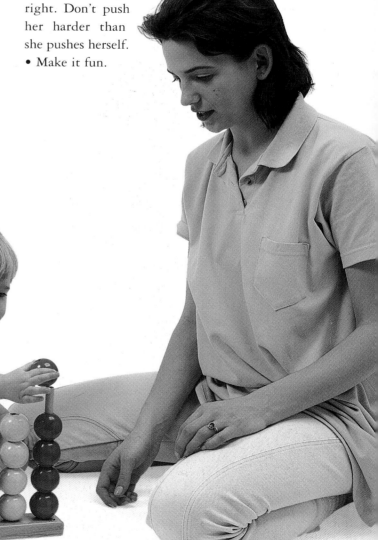

EVERYDAY CARE

The everyday physical care of an 18-month-old can be a balancing act between letting them assert themselves and take some control, and making sure that they're kept clean and healthy.

Toddlers tend to be quite determined little people. They have a growing awareness of their own bodies and often have strong views – expressed in no uncertain terms – about what's done to those bodies. They're also keen to do things for themselves.

GENERAL HYGIENE

Toddlers' hands get into everything, and then into their mouths, so you'll probably want to encourage your toddler in good hygiene practices.

One way of doing this is to get into the habit of washing your hands with her whenever hers need it, particularly before meals or snacks, or after playing in the garden or with pets. Once you've got her used to the idea of handwashing by soaping your hands and rubbing hers in yours, the time will come when she'll want to do it for herself. You can make this easier for her by providing a step which she can stand on to reach the basin by herself, though at first you'll probably still need to turn the taps on for her and help with rolling up sleeves. Be prepared for splashes – if not puddles – on the floor too.

BATHING YOUR TODDLER

Don't expect your toddler to keep clean. On the contrary, expect that she will get unbelievably grubby. Toddlers spend a lot of time on the floor, and they love mess. They're also not usually very skilled at eating and can end up with food in places where you didn't think it was possible for food to get.

Your toddler will probably be happier if you can accept that she's going to be grubby most of the time, and aren't constantly following her round with a damp flannel. Wipe off what needs to be wiped off to keep her comfortable and within the bounds of hygiene during the day, and leave the rest to an evening bath.

Most toddlers love baths. They like warm water and they enjoy water play, with floating and pouring toys. They may, though, object to being washed. You can get around this by using a mild bubble bath which will go some way towards removing the dirt. If your toddler has skin problems, your doctor may recommend a bath liquid that won't irritate her skin. If she doesn't like you washing her, she can wash herself, although make sure you squeeze the flannel out before letting her wash her face.

BATHTIME SAFETY

Although you won't need to hold your toddler in the bath, don't turn your back on her while she's in the water or leave her unattended. It's still possible for her to slip under the water. She may also try and turn on the hot tap or get hold of the soap and get it into her eyes.

Some toddlers are frightened of baths, however, which makes bathtime very distressing for everyone concerned. If this is the case for your toddler, you can try washing her in other ways – such as standing her up in a bowl of water and giving her an all-over wash, or letting her sit on the draining board and washing her from the sink, or standing her in the bath and spraying her, or letting her spray herself, with the shower attachment if you have one. When you want to get her back into the bath, getting in it with her, or providing some exciting new bath toys, can sometimes help overcome her reluctance.

HAIRWASHING

Many toddlers hate having their hair washed. But as an increasing number of substances seem to find their way into your toddler's hair, hairwashing is something that you can't always put off.

If hairwashing is a misery for your toddler, as well as for you, using a shampoo shield to keep the water off her face will sometimes help. Some toddlers will hold a flannel over their face to keep the water off if you give them one – though they probably won't want you to hold it there for them. Or they may be happier if they're allowed to wet their hair for themselves. Making funny shapes or Father Christmas beards with the shampoo lather and letting your toddler look at herself in a mirror can sometimes turn tears into smiles.

DENTAL CARE

For many toddlers, tooth-brushing is just an annoying distraction from the more fun things in life. Some parents try to encourage their toddlers in good tooth-brushing habits by making a game of it. Amanda makes it a joint exercise: 'First I brush my bottom teeth, then I brush Joe's. Then my top ones, then his.' Some toddlers like to brush their own teeth, though this needs to be followed up with adult brushing. Daniel takes it in turns with Eleanor: 'I brush my teeth with my toothbrush and Eleanor brushes her teeth with her toothbrush. Then I brush Eleanor's teeth with her toothbrush and she has a little go at mine. Seems only fair.'

Whatever method you use, your toddler's teeth need brushing twice a day, especially last thing at night.

Once your toddler has discovered that there are things called biscuits and sweets that other children have, you may find it more difficult to keep these out of her diet altogether. But her teeth will benefit if you can limit the quantity of sugary food that she has. Too many sweet drinks are best avoided too.

Taking your toddler to the dentist before she has a full set of first teeth might seem a bit premature, but introducing her early to the idea of going to the dentist can help make her less anxious about it later on. And it's possible for tooth decay to start before the age of two. Some parents get their child used to going to the dentist by taking her along when they go for a check-up themselves. Most dentists will be quite happy to let children have a go at sitting in the chair and to examine their teeth for them, if the child wants.

NAILS

If your toddler's fingernails aren't kept short, all manner of things – food, soil, playdough are among the more mentionable – can get under them. Toenails need to be kept short too, or shoes can be uncomfortable.

You'll need to cut your toddler's nails with round-ended scissors or nail clippers. You'll probably find it easiest to sit her on your lap, where you can hold her – relatively – still. Give her a toy, or sing to her. The rhyme 'This little piggy' was made for nail-cutting sessions.

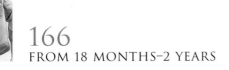
INDEPENDENCE AND DEPENDENCE

Life's tough for a toddler, wanting to do so much and unable to understand why she can't. And it's equally tough for those looking after her.

Toddlers can be maddening. One mum, Maria, called her husband home from work when their daughter Rebekah rubbed half a pot of Vaseline into her hair and the other half into the carpet, and Carrie remembers: 'We had one day with Harriet when she called the police in the morning, pooed all over my sister's bed at lunch-time, and then called the police on redial in the afternoon'. It's hard work, coping with a megalomaniac scientist, with a short memory and no self-control!

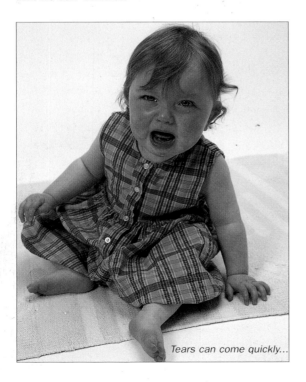

Tears can come quickly...

IN TRANSITION

So where did your happy, easy-going baby go and who is this querulous, defiant toddler, aggressively rejecting your help one minute, while crying and clinging to you the next? The fact is that your toddler is in transition between being a baby and becoming a child and it's a fragile and emotional time for everyone.

Your toddler's independence is often aggressive because he feels he has to push hard to escape his dependence on you, and when you try to help him he kicks all the harder because he doesn't want to slip back into babyhood again. In a way he is fighting for his life: a life of his own. But to get off to a good start he needs something stable to push against, and that just happens to be you.

For him, the world is an exciting place, full of amazing experiences and new things to play with. But excitement can easily topple over into fear. All it takes is for him to feel a little too far away from you, or to find himself pushed a little too fast towards an independence he doesn't feel, and he's terrified.

What your toddler wants is to be as physically close to you as possible – round your legs, in your arms, while insisting on psychological separation – insisting on doing it himself. The problem is, he doesn't have the skills to do some of the things he wants to do or the language to tell you what he wants. He wants to walk instead of ride in the buggy, but his short legs and fascination for every cigarette butt and crumpled tissue along the way drive you crazy. If you try to hurry him or put him back in the pushchair, the only way he has to express his frustration is through his behaviour. Which is why his reactions are often so extreme, and so sudden. Later, when he has a little more language, he'll be able to explain that he just wants to walk to the corner. And when his memory improves he'll be able to remember that last time he walked you didn't get to the park before it was time for tea and you had to go.

Following the guidelines below should make life with your toddler easier. Not easy, but easier. For the next year and a half, the bad days will be ones where you join in with the stamping and shouting. The good days will be those where you have the energy to remain open and

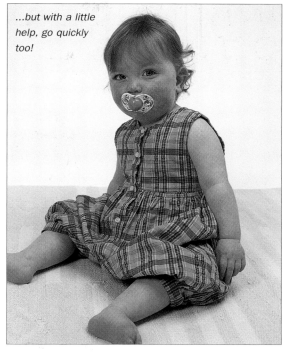

...but with a little help, go quickly too!

adaptable, ready to catch him if he can't handle the frustrations of life, while happy to see him striding out looking for new experiences.

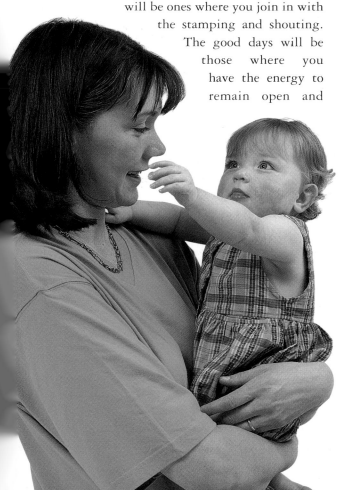

WHAT CAN YOU DO?

- don't baby him. He needs to make mistakes so he can learn from them
- try not to expect independence beyond his years. He needs to know that you love him for who he is now
- don't despair. All toddlers are as maddening, determined, loving, whiny and clingy as yours, believe it or not
- no need to feel guilty. Those intense feelings of love and hate you have for him are normal. Just compare notes with your friends
- slow down into 'baby time'. Does it really matter how long it takes?
- take a break. If you don't look after yourself, how can you look after him?

YOUR BABY
FROM 2–2½ YEARS

Many two-year-olds are passionate little people. Being caught in the transition between baby and child means that your toddler can be hard work and then delightful, both in the space of a few minutes.

Two-year-olds tend to approach problems head-on in all areas of their lives, whether it's pushing a wheelbarrow or dealing with bolshie parents. Working round something or being flexible is just not an option. Your toddler gives every impression of being unreasonable whereas, in fact, she is incapable of reason – quite a different thing.

Toddlers of this age are usually egocentric, unable to see anyone else's point of view or feelings. And this can make life tough for everyone concerned. But as happens across all areas of development – new abilities, new sensitivities, first appear in familiar situations. Your toddler may talk appropriately to the baby because she's used to seeing babies as different from other people. Or she may occasionally react to anger or tears in your family by trying to comfort the person who is upset. This may be the beginnings of empathy or it may be your toddler responding to the unhappiness she

experiences inside herself, by comforting her brother or sister as she would like to be comforted.

It's an emotional time. Although she'll start to play with other children at this stage, she won't be mature enough, on the whole, to understand that they have feelings too. She may snatch toys or hit and bite other children, cause a commotion and may even enjoy it all!

MEMORY IMPROVES

By two, toddlers' memories are much improved, especially for the things which interest them. They remember well which buttons to press to watch their video, and which cupboard to open to find the biscuits.

Toddlers of this age have the growing ability to imagine familiar objects when they are not there and to make plans about them. This is both wonderful and dreadful. Wonderful

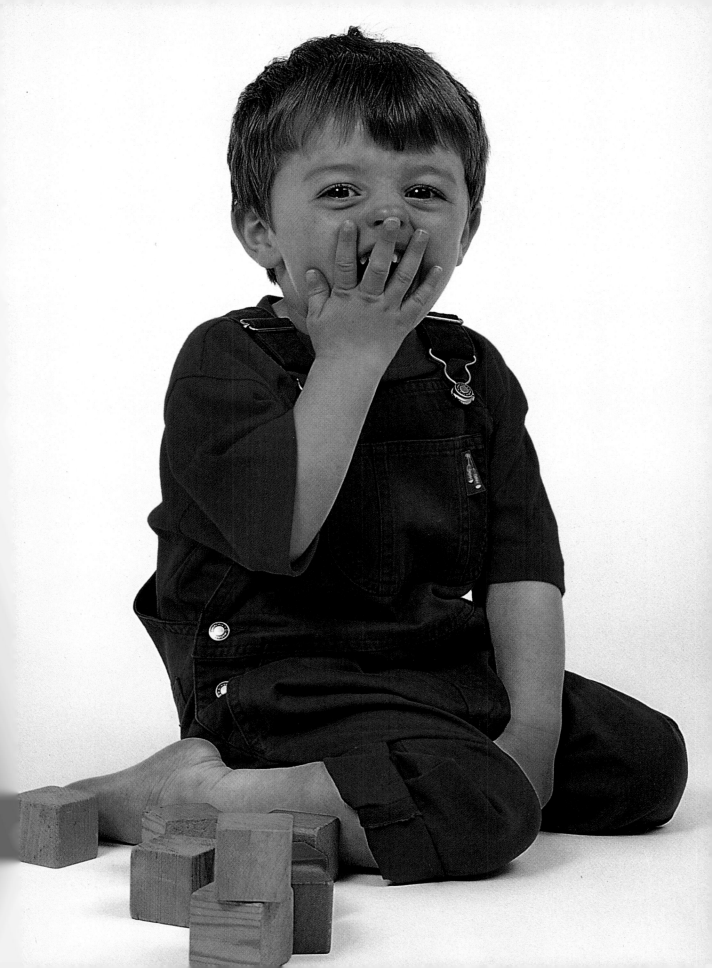

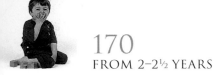

because it increases the potential for real relationships, which extend beyond one session at the toddler group – and games which can be left while she rushes to the loo and picked up again immediately afterwards. But dreadful because once she has imagined something, your toddler is unable to wait for that thing to happen. She has no concept of the day after tomorrow and in fact 'this afternoon' might well flummox her were it not for the explanatory term 'after lunch'.

LANGUAGE

Most toddlers are quick to pick up new words, and quick to integrate them into their monologues. By the time they reach two, many toddlers are able to use words to refer to things which they cannot see and most are good communicators – using a mix of spoken words, gestures and actions to express themselves. But your toddler still relies on you to do what comes naturally and speak to her in simple sentences, which are one step ahead of what she can produce herself: 'Please come and have your bath now.' 'Can you wash your face?'

In fact, toddlers themselves employ a special sort of language when they talk to a younger child (see 'motherese' page 188). For example, your toddler will use more repetitive and attention-eliciting words (like 'look!') when she talks to her younger brother or sister than she does when she talks to an adult.

Two-year-olds often have a good (though obviously infantile) sense of humour, laughing not only at those (by now) old jokes involving visual mistaken identity – pretending to brush your teeth with a hair-brush, for example – but also at verbal jokes too. Call her bed the bath or the car and you're bound to get a laugh.

Two-year-olds can walk and move much more quickly, although proper running usually doesn't come until around two-and-a-half. Suddenly everything seems to be within her grasp – no matter how high or far away you put it. All physical skills – walking, climbing, kicking and throwing a ball, stacking bricks, fitting, posting and drawing – need time and

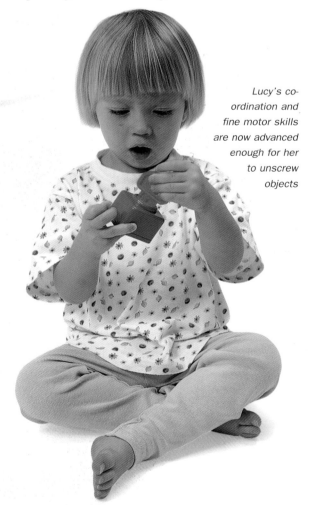

Lucy's co-ordination and fine motor skills are now advanced enough for her to unscrew objects

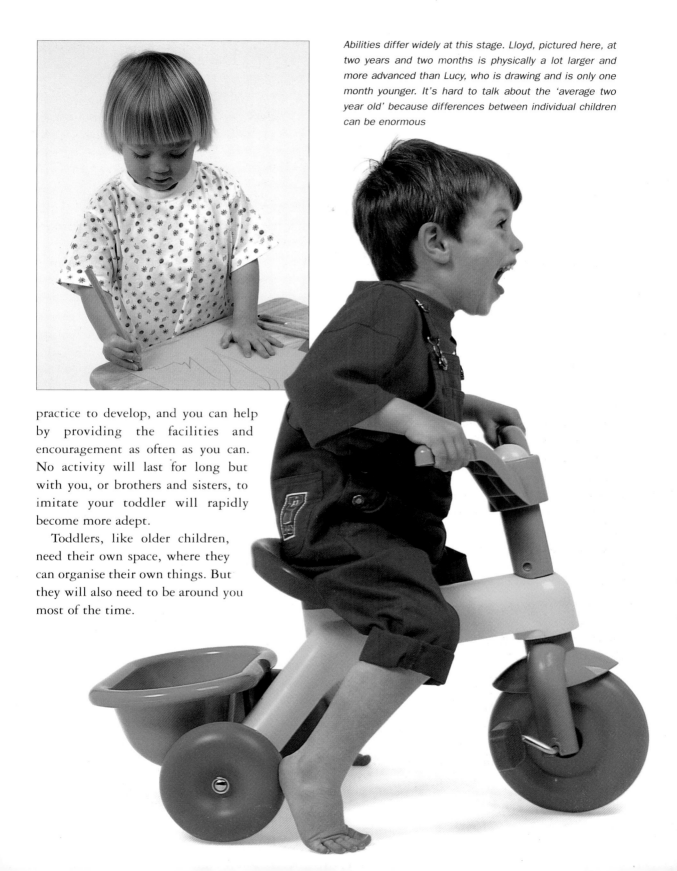

Abilities differ widely at this stage. Lloyd, pictured here, at two years and two months is physically a lot larger and more advanced than Lucy, who is drawing and is only one month younger. It's hard to talk about the 'average two year old' because differences between individual children can be enormous

practice to develop, and you can help by providing the facilities and encouragement as often as you can. No activity will last for long but with you, or brothers and sisters, to imitate your toddler will rapidly become more adept.

Toddlers, like older children, need their own space, where they can organise their own things. But they will also need to be around you most of the time.

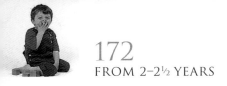

DIARY OF A TWO-YEAR-OLD

Michael is two years old. He goes to nursery every morning while his mother, Pippa, works from home. Rob, his father, is out at work during the day.

6am

Michael wakes up and goes into his parents' bed. He is now sleeping in a bed, so he can get up by himself. His nappy – which now usually stays dry all night – is taken off and he uses the potty. Michael is still in nappies, but Pippa takes him to use the potty several times during the day and he is starting to ask for it himself. He is *very* proud of himself for using it.

Pippa or Rob reads Michael a story in their bed, then he goes back to his bedroom and plays on his own for a while. Although he enjoys playing with his parents, he's also happy to entertain himself. He loves to build things – especially aeroplanes – with Duplo or Sticklebricks.

7am

Pippa gets up and dressed, then dresses Michael. Pippa usually chooses what he will wear, although he is very particular about his shoes and socks. He likes to try and do his buttons up and to put his shoes on. 'I smart,' he says.

7.45am

Michael helps Pippa make breakfast. He pours the milk into his cereal – and has now learnt when to stop pouring – and likes to butter his toast all by himself. He has outgrown his highchair, so he eats his breakfast sitting on a chair at the table. He is now able to feed himself using a fork and a spoon, and is quite co-ordinated about it.

8.30am

Another visit to the potty, then off to nursery.

12.45pm

Pippa collects Michael from nursery, where he has had his lunch. He has a bottle of milk, then goes for a nap.

3pm

Michael wakes up or Pippa wakes him and he uses the potty. Then it's 'Play, Mummy'. Michael likes to use his hands and his favourite activities involve building or making things, or drawing. When it's fine, he plays in his sandpit in the garden, or on his swing or his tricycle, while Pippa does gardening. He likes to help and especially enjoys digging for worms. Recently he has begun to engage in imaginative play. He has a 'house' in a hollow tree trunk in the garden where he makes imaginary cups of tea

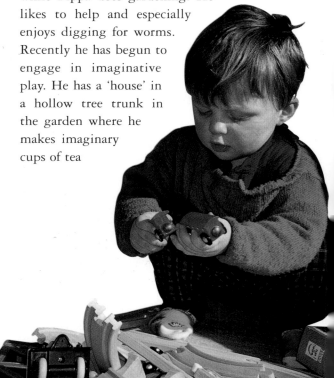

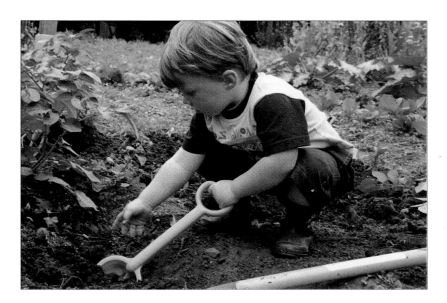

6.45pm
Bathtime with Daddy.

7.15pm
Time to wind down and quietly do jigsaw puzzles or read books. Michael particularly likes books which have realistic pictures of animals, or of machines like aeroplanes, fire engines or tractors. He has a bottle of milk to help relax him for bed.

and sandwiches for Pippa or for his favourite teddies. Sometimes he likes to involve Pippa in this pretend play, but other times he prefers to play on his own. Sometimes instead of playing, Michael helps Pippa to bake, or they go to the park, or they see friends, including some that Pippa made at her NCT antenatal class.

4pm
Time for a cup of tea and a snack. Michael enjoys the ritual of making the tea and pouring it out. He likes to have the same thing to drink as Pippa.

After tea, Michael continues playing. If he's playing on his own, he becomes very absorbed in what he's doing, and doesn't like to be interrupted. 'I busy. I fine,' he says, if Pippa calls him to do something else. Being interrupted from his activities is the main thing that makes him upset.

6pm
Michael has his supper. Rob often comes home at this time, so he sits with Michael while he has his supper and then plays with him till bathtime.

7.45pm
Bedtime. Pippa sits on a chair in Michael's bedroom and they sing a few songs. Although he used to be happy to go to sleep on his own, at the moment, Michael likes Pippa to stay in the room until he's asleep. He tends to wake once most nights and to call out for Pippa, but he goes back to sleep again quickly.

8pm
Michael is usually asleep. Pippa and Rob have time together having supper and catching up on the day, or reading or watching television. 'We hardly ever go out,' says Pippa. 'I think we've been to the cinema about three times in the last two years! We just like being at home.'

Pippa loves being involved in Michael's activities. 'I enjoy playing with him and watching him learn,' she says. 'I love his enthusiasm and the way he's so excited about everything.' She's apprehensive about the future, though. 'I worry about him going out into the world.' But for now, she lets herself be guided by Michael. 'I try not to demand too much of him and to let him develop at his own rate.'

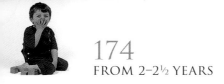

LANGUAGE AT TWO YEARS

Between two and two-and-a-half years old, toddlers eventually become more like adults in their use of language, although their pronunciation is still very childlike.

Two-year-olds are great talkers and most can produce all the vowel sounds. With the consonants, though, many find it easier to use the ones that are produced at the front of the mouth, saying 'tuddle' instead of 'cuddle'. Toddlers often omit consonants at the ends of words which makes it hard to understand them.

When he is just two your toddler may refer to himself by name, as in 'Joe do it' or 'Adam fall down'. But before he is two-and-a-half he will have learnt to say 'me' and probably 'I' as well. He may use 200 words or more, although he will probably understand around one thousand.

Some of these words will be descriptions like 'good', 'bad', 'hard', 'dirty' or 'nice'.

When your toddler first started to speak he used words to label things he could see. Now he will begin to use those words to talk about different times and places, to talk about his desires. But his desires run ahead of his knowledge of words. Most two-year-olds usually still talk in the present tense even about things from the past or the future. For example, 'Ben go party' could refer to a party which happened last week, is happening now or is only a wish for the future.

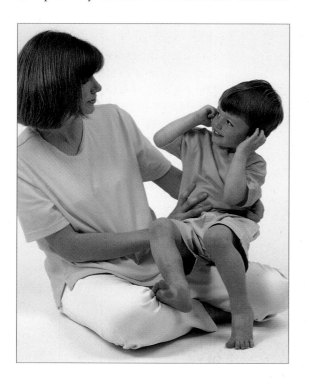

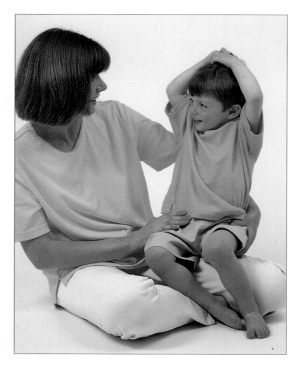

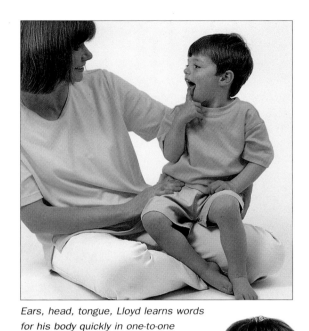

Ears, head, tongue, Lloyd learns words
for his body quickly in one-to-one
conversation with
his mother

PARROTING

At this age toddlers listen attentively when talked to and blatantly eavesdrop other peoples' conversations as well, collecting new words to use. Sometimes your toddler will parrot new words that take his fancy then and there, and other times he will play with them later, working them into the long incomprehensible monologues he uses when he plays. Often you will hear your toddler repeating a scolding or an instruction as he plays, trying to learn the script. It can be a humbling experience hearing your own words from your child as he ticks off his teddy for getting out of bed or not eating his plastic fishfinger tea. ('You're a naughty teddy' and on and on!)

SECOND LANGUAGE

If yours is a two-language family, your children will learn to understand and speak both languages – a definite advantage in later life. It's easiest if each parent always addresses the child in his or her own first language; the child will reserve that particular way of speaking for that adult and gradually become fluent.

PHYSICAL SKILLS

Toddlers are extremely busy people and a child at this stage can get up to all sorts of mischief.

Physical changes in his legs and feet will now help your two-year-old boost his physical skills. Ankles and knees are becoming more flexible, legs longer, less chubby and more muscular, and flat feet develop arches. This means your toddler will be busy learning how to run safely and to side-step, to walk up and down stairs (albeit with two feet on each step initially), to stand easily from squatting – while keeping a firm grip on whichever toy he thinks might be snatched away by another toddler – and to walk backwards, often while pulling the handle of a large wheeled toy.

Your two-year-old is also pretty good with his hands. He can open, close, twist and push all sorts of doors, sweets, boxes, telephones, remote control units and other electronic gadgets. Coupled with his ability to climb as well as his newly

'The other day Callum was just too clever for his own good. He watched me put all of the shopping away and then, because he knew I would say "no" he dragged a chair in from the lounge, climbed up and onto the counter and helped himself to a biscuit.'

developing ability to plan ahead, your toddler's manual dexterity can be devastating.

Your toddler may hold his pencil or paintbrush in his fist or, if you show him how, he may be able to move towards a proper writers' three-finger or 'tripod' grip. He'll also copy you if you draw a circle. Overall, he'll be taking more interest in the marks he makes.

Gradually he'll learn to hold the paper steady with one hand as he draws with the other and to name his circle, dot and line creations as 'a cat' or 'mummy' (though it may be hard for you to see the difference). By now he'll probably prefer to use one hand rather than the other.

GETTING SORTED

Toddlers are beginning to get interested in different categories of things. Sort out the contents of her underwear drawer into socks, pants, vests. Pasta shapes, bricks, simple puzzles, stacking rings or shape sorters are all good alternatives to sorting underwear if you want to develop hand–eye co-ordination and control of the small muscles in the hand.

Improved balance and

A JUMP START
Physical changes to your toddler's body mean that he may soon be able to jump from the lowest step, two feet at a time. It's a task that takes great co-ordination as he has to jump up as well as out. But if it's something he wants to do, he will practise repeatedly. At first his legs will be rigid as he lands, but gradually he'll learn to bend his knees to soften the impact, and to use his arms to help him balance and not fall over.

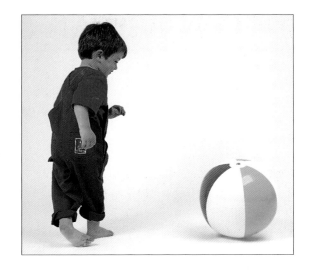

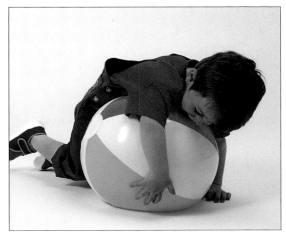

co-ordination mean that some toddlers now start to rock their bodies or to move their feet in time to music, while others can sit on a tricycle and propel themselves forward by pushing with their feet – although it may take a year or so before their legs are strong enough, and their co-ordination and balance good enough to start to use the pedals.

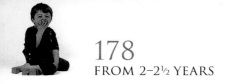
TODDLER TANTRUMS

Don't expect your two-year-old to share her toys or think of others.
At this stage, toddlers think only of themselves. They can't help it.

Your toddler has yet to understand that other people are people in the same way that she is – thinking, feeling and sociable. Concepts like 'waiting', 'sharing', 'helping' and 'being reasonable' are just so many words. The only thing that motivates her is doing what she wants. Of course, there will be times when your toddler is kind or reasonable or does share, but it will be because she happens to want to do whatever it was that seems kind or reasonable to you. She wants what she wants and when you say 'no', it's hard work for her to cope.

ALLOWING CHOICE

At this all-or-nothing stage, your toddler will find making a choice difficult because it means she won't be able to have both options at once. She does want to do things for herself, though, so allow her to choose wherever possible.

It will help if you present her with no-lose choices, where whatever she chooses is something nice, and she won't wish she'd done the other thing. Ask: 'Do you want to go on the slide or the swing first?' for example.

Allow real choices – 'Either you eat it or you go hungry' is not a choice; 'Do you want yoghurt, fruit or both?' is.

Limit your child's choice – too much is confusing. Dozens of ice cream flavours may be wonderfully exciting for teenagers, but your toddler may be happier if you just offer him chocolate or vanilla.

TERRIBLE TWOS

But no matter how great a parent you are, tantrums are still part of the toddler job description. They get grouchy, of course, when they're tired or hungry or over-excited, and part of your job is not to let that happen but then again, tantrums can blow up out of nowhere, in spite of your best efforts.

COPING WITH TANTRUMS

Keep as calm as you can and try not to get angry – she may be scared by the control she has over you and by the force of her anger. Once you've

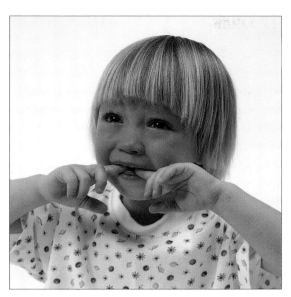

said 'no' don't give in – giving in signals to your child that if she holds out long enough she'll get what she wants. Instead, decide on a plan of action and stick to it. Either ignore the tantrum, but stay near to her, or hold her firmly (without hurting her) until she is all cried out.

Keep your explanations until after the tantrum is over, and you've made friends again – even if she can hear you above her cries she won't understand you.

Do not reward her tantrum. Do give her a cuddle afterwards but save it for a little later, or she may feel that the cuddle is her reward. Then give yourself time to cool off – you deserve it.

Keep a note of things that trigger tantrums and try to avoid these in the future.

Your calm and loving response will show her that you can help her to cope with her frustration and anger. Gradually she will feel safe expressing negative emotions while learning how to cope with them herself. As your toddler becomes better at expressing herself, her tantrums should subside. Soon there will come a day when she can calmly tell you what it is that she wants, without drumming her heels and screaming.

TODDLER SAFETY

- Turn pan-handles towards the back. Some parents like to fit a cooker guard, but don't rely on it as a way of keeping hands off.
- Put protectors on the corners of low tables.
- Fit safety glass, or buy special film in D-I-Y shops to cover low windows or glass doors.
- Put safety catches on your doors to stop little fingers getting crushed.
- Make sure your furniture is arranged to limit potentially dangerous climbing opportunities.
- See that free-standing bookcases or cupboards can't be pulled over and store toys where he won't climb to get them.
- Don't leave objects lying around on stairs.
- No running in socks on polished floors.
- Fasten down any loose flooring.
- Ensure that he can't open the front door.
- Make sure that doors can't be locked from the inside, or move locks up, out of reach.
- Turn the hot water temperature down to 54°C (130°F) or less, to avoid scalding.
- Fit safety catches on windows.
- Lock garden sheds.
- Cover water butts.
- Cover ponds or fence off – better still, fill them in for a year or two. Toddlers can easily drown in garden ponds, and they do.
- Make sure that there are no escape routes from the garden, including holes in hedges. Fit safety catches to gates.
- Teach your child not to eat berries.
- Keep a First Aid kit handy and know what to do in an emergency.

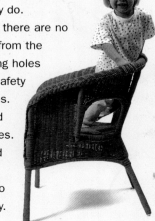

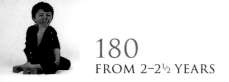

PLAY AT TWO YEARS

Most toddlers of this age can stick to one activity for a maximum of 12 minutes. So you'll need to have a lot of options available because each time he finishes one game, he may need a bit of help getting started with the next.

Children play because it is fun. And part of the fun is the way in which play allows your toddler increased mastery over his toys and himself. What he needs from you are well organised and accessible toys, time for him to play and your help, guidance and inspiration when needed.

Your toddler needs to take the lead in the games he plays with you. Playing in the way that he chooses will give him essential practice in self-direction and self-confidence – two important life skills. Play can also help your toddler come to terms with frightening experiences – real or imagined.

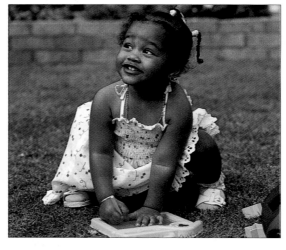

IMAGINATIVE PLAY

Your toddler will continue to imitate as before. But now some of his imitations will be more imaginative. For example, he'll pretend to feed himself with an empty spoon scooping from an empty bowl, or to offer his favoured toy a bite of his biscuit. There is an element of originality in his play. Your toddler has seen that sort of activity many times before, using just such tools but he may never have seen a toy being fed, or someone eating from an empty bowl.

At about this age, toddlers also begin to imitate each other as well as important adults around them. Not many toddlers yet play with each other, but they can begin to play alongside, often keeping a running commentary on the state of play as they go. Each time one toddler first does something different, the other toddlers are likely to try it too. If the dolls are all being fed and one has to have a little wind brought up, it's uncanny how rapidly that wind will spread from one doll to the other.

Your toddler will probably watch other children at play, and may even join in for a few minutes. But playing with others

SHARING WITH OTHERS

It's probably just as well that toddlers of this age play alongside each other most of the time, because when they play together about half the time they end up squabbling – often over one particular toy and sometimes even when there are two of them available.

Sharing is a hard lesson to learn. Just occasionally your toddler will accept the need to take turns – a first step on the way to real sharing, where each child uses the whatever-it-is until they no longer need it and then offers it to the other child – who meanwhile hovers and waits more-or-less-patiently for his turn.

requires a degree of co-operation and an ability to plan ahead that your toddler just doesn't have yet, and he will quickly revert to his solitary game where he can control what happens, taking with him some of the ideas from the other children's games.

So, your toddler is gaining a better sense of himself psychologically. At the same time he's developing a better sense of himself physically too. Playing with these new awarenesses is the best way for him to understand them better. So, just as he plays with his sense of self through imitation and make-believe, so he plays with his sense of his body through new games like hide-and-seek. He's learnt how big he is in relation to bits of furniture but he won't be able to hide effectively until he is about four years old when he will finally understand that another person does not see what he does. For now, when asked to hide, he may well stand in full view and cover his own eyes, believing that if he can't see you, you can't see him. At this age he may also forget, in his excitement who is hiding and who

is seeking. Getting to grips with different roles and perspectives takes a long time.

Your toddler is just as likely to play with the loo brush as his pull-along caterpillar. To him, everyday objects are just as fascinating as the toys you buy. And in terms of developing physical, mental, manipulative and social skills they may well be equally useful. As one mother says, 'I've had to make all my kitchen drawers redundant because Rowan (15 months) has learnt how to climb into the bottom one and then pull everything out of the top two!'

It's up to you to decide what is off-limits — but don't expect your toddler to remember from one hour to the next where you have set the boundaries.

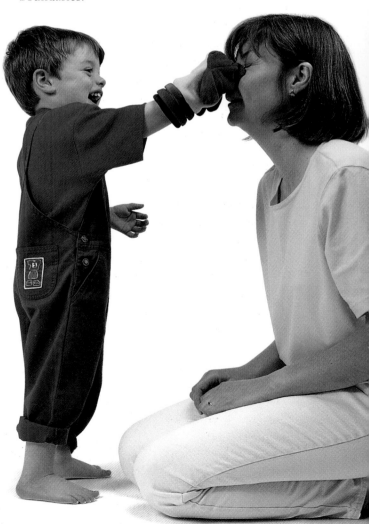

YOUR BABY FROM 2½–3 YEARS

By the age of two and a half most toddlers have a sense of their body image and most know whether they are a boy or a girl. They begin to use the words 'mine' and 'I' and to become definite in their desires.

For all their assertions, toddlers need frequent reassurance that they are valued and loved. Your toddler will need you to acknowledge all her achievements and commiserate with her failures. Saying 'never mind' when the paint has spilt over her picture suggests that the picture isn't important. Acknowledging that she is upset may help her to feel valued and ultimately to put away her tears and move on to a fresh piece of paper and another picture.

PROMISES, PROMISES

Your toddler often looks and sounds older than she really is. She may well use words which she doesn't understand, but which sound plausible. Words like 'promise'. At this age it's probably better not to ask her to promise anything because she's not in a position to be able to faithfully keep one. She wants to but when it comes to the point she may be swayed by circumstances which are just too pressing to ignore. When you've yet to discover who you are, it's difficult to say whether you will or you won't do something or other.

Your toddler probably enjoys make-believe by now. Make-believe play involves not just copying behaviour, but being able to do it without having anyone to copy at the time, and often without the original tools available either. It's a quantum leap in your toddler's ability, and depends on improved memory, and extended powers of concentration. Make-believe games initially involve playing roles which are familiar to your toddler. Mums and babies or mums and dads are early favourites. But later on superheroes, doctors and nurses, dentists, and train drivers may all have cameo parts, depending on your child's experiences.

Children learn a lot by playing out these different roles. Make-believe is also useful in

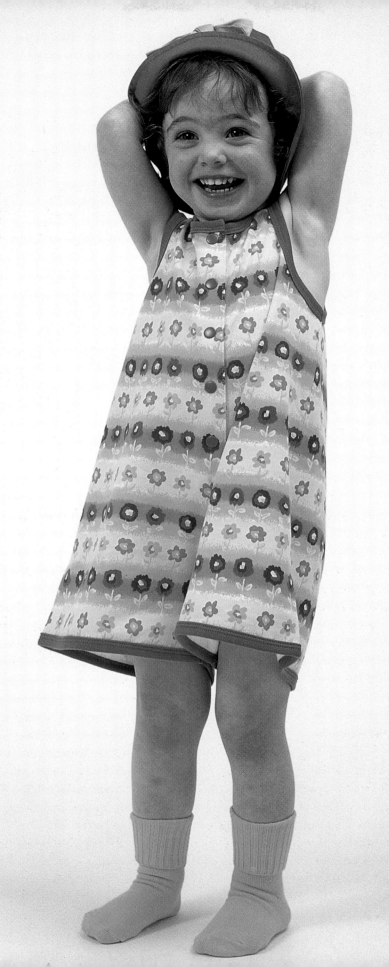

times of stress – moving house, the arrival of a new sibling, the death of someone loved, because it helps your toddler to come to terms with the experience. Toddlers who act out such events in their games should be allowed to do so unchecked, so that the fear can be made less frightening. Many toddlers become so engrossed in make-believe play with a particular character that they seem to spend most of the day in role. There are usually at least two or three Batmans or princesses at the park, fighting off baddies on the swings or being rescued from the climbing frame.

A SENSE OF SELF

Your toddler's newfound ability to make believe is part of her developing sense of other people. By playing with the idea of different points of view – playing at mums and babies for example

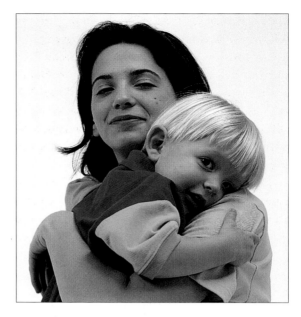

– your toddler develops a sense of others, and at the same time, a sense of herself.

Toddlers can only get a clearer idea of themselves by mixing with other people and copying what those people do: trying on for size different ways of behaving.

Your toddler is also trying on for size different ways of behaving when she begins to shout to get attention or to smile sweetly for a second helping. How you respond to these different identities defines how your toddler will feel about herself. The toddler who pushes others does not know that this is dangerous, and she will not know unless she is told. But if she is told off by being pushed back, she will only learn that push leads to shove, not that she shouldn't do it. The toddler whose parents show her that the other child cried when she was pushed and that a cuddle might help, will have learnt that pushing is wrong but that she can make things better, if she wants.

If you ask your toddler to draw a picture she will probably make large sweeping movements, but when asked to write she will make smaller, staccato marks on the page. Already, even before she recognises a single word, your toddler will see the difference between drawing and writing. 'When Thomas (31 months) sees writing, he asks, "What does that say?" He knows that the writing has meaning.'

Your child is inventing language as she speaks. At this age finding out new and exciting things and talking about them are one and the same thing: she sees something amazing and she

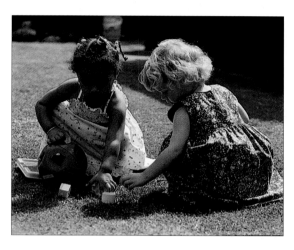

lets you know. The problem for your social life is that your toddler discovers new things hundreds of times a day.

As language ability grows, so concepts are now developing – concepts of quantity, for example, such as 'one' or 'many'. This is a good time to start teaching numbers. At lunch-time you could sit a teddy up at the table and let your toddler lay a place for herself, one for you and one for teddy. By giving each person a place setting and putting out cutlery, she will be starting basic maths.

Comparisons are a new idea, too. As you unpack the shopping, ask her to compare sizes between, say, potatoes. Teach 'bigger than' and 'smaller than' (making the difference in size very obvious at first to avoid confusion). Ask her to give you one tin to put on the shelf, then two tins. See if she can understand the concepts 'empty' and 'full'. Give her simple instructions to follow, such as 'please put the apples in the fruit bowl' or 'please fetch me that box of cornflakes'. She will enjoy being your little helper and (if you're not in a hurry) you'll probably have fun too. If you're really getting into it, you could let her help you do some cooking. Break down the work into manageable tasks and she'll feel really proud of herself.

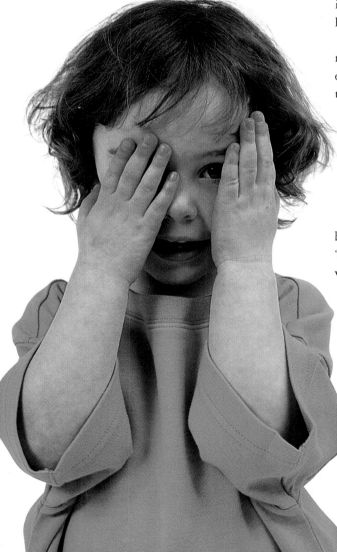

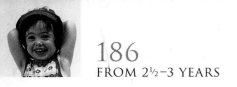

DIARY OF 2½-YEAR-OLD TWINS

Samuel and Jacob are twins. Their mother, Cathleen, doesn't have a job outside the home. Their father, Ian, works shifts, so is at home at different times on different days.

Cathleen is finding Samuel and Jacob quite challenging at the moment: 'They're pushing barriers, always trying to see how far they can go.' But she also finds their developing language and mental abilities fascinating: 'Sometimes I think, "now how on earth did they know that?" They're amazing.'

6.30am

Jacob is usually the first to wake up. He gets out of bed and goes into his parents' bedroom, so they're soon awake too. They generally manage to have a little while longer in bed, though, while Jacob amuses himself with things in their room.

7am

Cathleen gets up and goes downstairs with Jacob. He has a drink of milk and Cathleen encourages him to play quietly with his toys or to watch television for a while. 'He's on the go all day, so I try not to let him get started too early,' she says.

7.30am

Samuel wakes up and Cathleen brings him downstairs for a drink too. Then she begins the process of getting the twins dressed. This can be quite a struggle, as although Cathleen likes the boys to be dressed before breakfast, they see no reason at all to get out of their pyjamas.

8.30am

Cathleen takes a relaxed approach to breakfast, and Samuel and Jacob often have some toast and milk in the living room, rather than sitting up at the table. They'll have their breakfast in between short bursts of playing or watching television. 'They never seem to do anything for more than about five minutes,' says Cathleen. 'Their concentration span is very short.'

9.30am

Samuel and Jacob have finished their breakfast, and Cathleen decides what to do for the morning. Sometimes they go to the park with their bikes, or they visit Cathleen's parents who live nearby, or they go shopping. Samuel and Jacob like being outside, so they particularly enjoy the park. Cathleen finds that when they're playing outside, they do more together and are less competitive with each other than when they're indoors. They also enjoy meeting other children in the park. Another favourite activity is pretending that the bark chips around the play equipment are food, and putting them to their mouths as if they're eating them. 'They know they're not supposed to put them in their mouths. They do it to tease me,' says Cathleen.

12noon

If they've been out, Cathleen tries to be home by noon so that Samuel and Jacob can have a

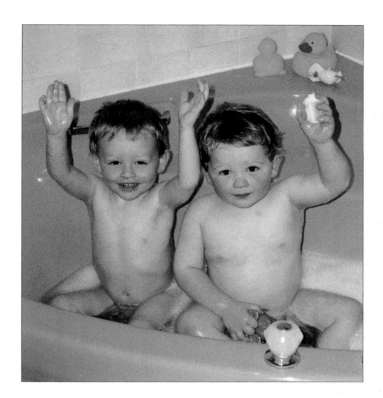

nap for an hour or two. If she's had a disturbed night – the twins aren't good sleepers – Cathleen uses this time to rest herself. Otherwise she catches up on things she finds it difficult to do when the boys are awake.

2pm

Lunchtime. If Ian is at home, they all have a hot meal together, otherwise they may have a cold lunch. Ian likes experimenting with different foods, and Samuel and Jacob always like to have a taste of what he's having, if it's something different.

2.30pm

If they've been out in the morning, Cathleen, Samuel and Jacob usually stay at home in the afternoon. Samuel and Jacob tend to fight quite a lot when they're indoors, so Cathleen encourages them to play outside with their cars, or on their bikes. They also like water play and

playing with bubbles. If Ian is at home, they may all go out on family errands. Cathleen has found that when they go out, getting Samuel and Jacob into their car seats or pushchair is much easier if she allows them to climb in on their own. 'They like to be independent.'

5pm

Time to start winding down for the end of the day. Cathleen encourages Samuel and Jacob to play quietly, doing puzzles or looking at books or comics.

6pm

Teatime, followed by more quiet play until it's time to get ready for bed.

7pm

Bathtime. Samuel and Jacob get themselves undressed and climb into the bath themselves. They have great fun squirting water at each other and splashing it all over the floor.

7.45pm

Samuel and Jacob get into bed and Cathleen reads them stories. They have a drink, then put the beakers and the books away themselves. One of them turns the light off – then Cathleen puts it on again so that the other one can turn it off too.

Neither Samuel nor Jacob tends to settle very well, so Cathleen usually stays in the room until they've gone to sleep. For her, this is a time to relax and unwind and, as she puts it, 'to think my own thoughts', which she doesn't have much time for during the day.

9pm

Both boys are usually asleep.

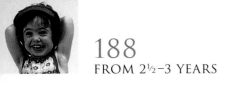

LANGUAGE AT 2½

Toddlers learn to talk at widely differing times – some will be using well over 200 words by now, and others will have only just begun to name things.

Those toddlers with more words will probably now be demanding to know 'what' and 'who' about everything and everyone, sometimes embarrassingly loudly. Early talkers are often those who've had a lot of one-to-one conversation with an adult. Boys, however, do tend to talk a little later than girls. This is probably because most boys focus on activities and most girls on relationships, and it's just impossible to have a relationship with someone unless you've told them your name, shown them your doll, and giggled together!

Many toddlers get so excited by their ability to share their experiences that they stutter. You can help by calmly repeating the sentence that you think he wants to say, and then acting on it. Don't make an issue of it. It will probably pass.

BAA BAA BLACK SHEEP

Toddlers love repetition, and nursery rhymes and simple stories fit the bill perfectly. Many toddlers gleefully choose the same story over and over again until either the book or their parent expires. 'Last week I was really wicked. I told Hetty (32 months) that "Each, Peach, Pear, Plum" was a library book and we had to take it back. I just couldn't stand reading it again.

'Poor Hetty. I've promised myself I'll get it back from "the library" at the back of my wardrobe when I'm feeling stronger.'

'MOTHERESE'

You will probably find that, almost without realising it, you employ a special way of talking to your toddler. Psychologists have studied this and come up with the name 'motherese' to describe it, although it's

'Evette's (35 months) favourite questions are "What is that person doing?" And "What does this or that animal like to eat?" She's fascinated by what they eat so it's "Mummy, what does an elephant eat?" And "Mummy, what does a bat eat?" I try to answer her if I can.'

not confined to mothers alone. Everyone who talks to children a lot, automatically adjusts the level of speech they use to the child's understanding.

Motherese is characterised by short, simple sentences which are spoken very slowly and clearly. Words are chosen with care so that each refers to something concrete and visible and that is sure to attract interest. Words are often repeated. For example, 'Look at that cat. It's a big cat.' Parents look at the things they are referring to and rarely talk about anything that's abstract or absent. Children even copy this way of talking when they're 'playing mummies and daddies'.

It has been known for mothers, who have spent all day talking motherese to their toddlers to find themselves continuing in that mode at, say, an adults' evening dinner party. 'Look at that table. What a lovely table!' etc.

INVENTING LANGUAGE

Your toddler is working hard on his language. He's busy learning the rules of talking about things from the past and the future. Often he applies the rules too widely: he's heard you use '-ed' on the ends of words about the past, so he says 'I comed in,' or 'I hurted my knee.'

He's heard you add an 's' to make a noun plural so he talks about 'foots' or 'sheeps'. He may even add an 's' to a word that is already plural because he hardly ever hears the singular and say, 'I putted on my shoeses.' He's yet to learn that the English language can trip him up just as easily as his own feet.

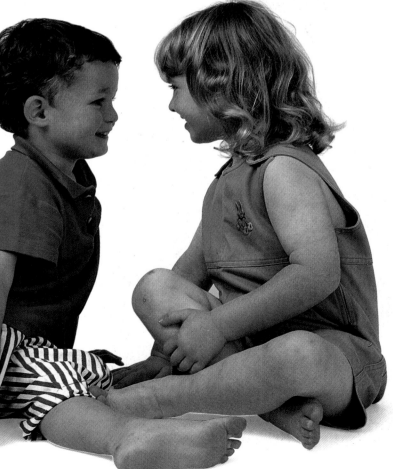

GETTING DRESSED

At two-and-a-half some toddlers are ready for the challenge of dressing themselves and are delighted when they succeed. On the other hand, some toddlers would rather not waste their precious time struggling with something which you can obviously do so much better.

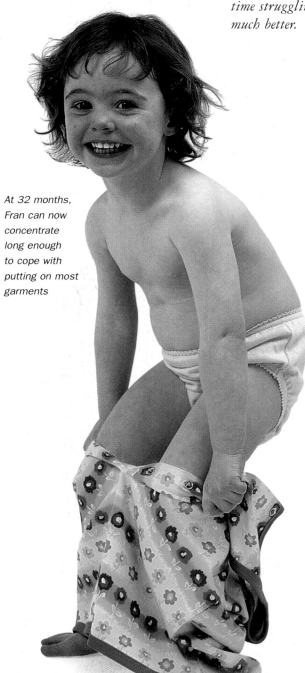

At 32 months, Fran can now concentrate long enough to cope with putting on most garments

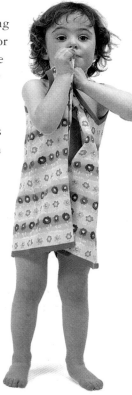

It's definitely worth buying clothes which will be easy for your toddler to put on and take off by themselves. Look for elasticated, loose-fitting and stretchy clothes, so that your child has as large a hole as possible to point her toe, arm or head at. Try to avoid tiny buttons or poppers or inaccessible zips.

At this age, things still come off easier than they go on. A year ago your toddler would probably have been able to remove his shoes, socks and hat, and by now he will be able to remove all his clothes, sometimes at wildly inappropriate times. Some children seem to

'Rebekah (27 months) can take her clothes off, but putting them on is something else. She's OK with socks, trousers and shoes but cannot manage sleeves yet. One morning I found her with her head and arm through the neck of her pyjamas, the other arm in one sleeve and one sleeve flapping – I think she'd been practising.'

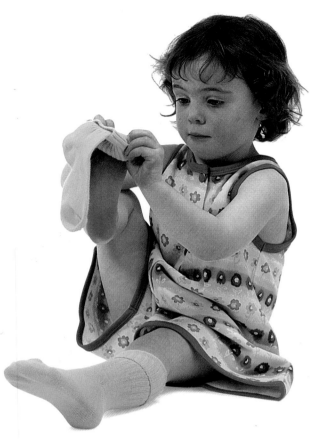

'Jonathan is becoming a monster with clothes. The other day I went into the nursery where he'd been having a nap and he was standing in bed, starkers – trousers, T-shirt and nappy all on the floor.'

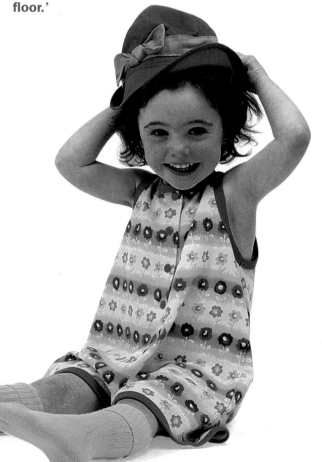

have an aversion to wearing clothes. 'I'm sure people think I'm an abusive mother. When we go out there's me in a shirt, two jumpers and David's old jacket and Adam (32 months) is wearing a T-shirt. As soon as I put anything on he takes it off again. He just doesn't seem to feel the cold.'

By the age of three, most children are able to dress and undress themselves in pull-on clothes. Of course, dressing yourself doesn't come all at once, some garments are easier than others. Six months ago, your toddler may have been happy to slip her feet into shoes, and plop a hat on her head, especially when both items were yours and she could play at being 'mummy' or 'daddy'. But tying up those shoes, especially if they are lace-ups, often doesn't happen until later – much later. You're better off sticking to Velcro until your toddler has laces all tied up.

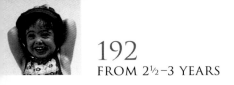

OUT OF NAPPIES

Maybe because of the expense and the effort involved, or maybe because no one really likes changing nappies, most parents eagerly look forward to the day when their child starts using a potty.

Children give up wearing nappies in their own time. When they're ready to do so, you can help them, but you can't do anything to make them ready any sooner – it depends entirely on the child's physical maturity. It can be galling to have your child still in nappies when everyone else's seems to be happily using the potty, but it's unlikely to be because of anything you're doing wrong – his body just isn't quite ready yet.

For a child to be able to use a potty, he needs to have conscious control over his bladder and bowel. In other words, he needs to be able to recognise the signs that he needs to do a wee or a poo (these are the words most commonly used with British children) and to be able to hold on until he's in the right place to do so.

GAINING CONTROL

Most children gain control somewhere between 18 and 36 months, with boys generally taking a little longer than girls. If you wait until you see signs that your child may be developing control, the process of getting him to use the potty can be relatively quick and painless. If you start too soon, it'll take longer and there'll be more accidents along the way. Look for these signs:

• He tells you that he's done a wee or a poo, or points to his nappy.

• He has longer intervals between wet nappies and may stay dry after a nap.

• He does poos at regular times.

• He can pull his clothes up and down by himself.

• He understands simple instructions.

INTRODUCING A POTTY

Many parents get a potty to have in the house for days – or even weeks – before they suggest that their child use it. Some show it to their child and explain what it's for. Others just leave it lying around for their child to discover by himself. Some children are very interested in the potty, as Claire found: 'Matthew was very excited when we got the potty because he'd seen children at nursery using one. He sat on it straight away.' Others aren't: 'Abigail didn't want to know at first. Then after a while I found her sitting her teddy on it and telling him what it was for, so she obviously had the idea.'

To get your toddler used to the idea of using the potty, try letting him sit on it clothed for a few days. Then encourage him to sit on it without a nappy, maybe just after you've taken a dirty nappy off. When he's got used to sitting without a nappy, you can suggest he take his nappy off and sits on the potty after a meal. He might just do something, although at this stage it will probably be more by luck than judgement. But if you give him lots of praise, that may encourage him to try a repeat performance.

If at any point he refuses to sit on the potty, try not to be cross with him, even though you may be feeling disappointed or infuriated.

Parents aren't saints, though this is a time when showing the patience of a saint is to your own advantage in the long run.

ENCOURAGEMENT

- Be relaxed about it.
- Give him lots of praise.
- Put him in clothes that are easy for him to remove.
- Have more than one potty in different parts of the house so that he doesn't have far to go.
- In the early stages, let him go without nappies or pants. This is obviously easier in the summer than in mid-January.
- Give him a small reward for using the potty (many parents do, giving something like a chocolate drop, though often feel that they probably shouldn't).

Try to avoid:
- Badgering him or forcing him to sit on it.
- Showing disgust at potty contents.
- Getting cross with accidents.
- Making him wait when he's asked for the potty.
- Introducing the potty at a time when other changes are going on in his life – such as a new baby, or moving house, or going on holiday.

Potty practicalities
- Put a piece of loo paper in the bottom of the potty to make it easier to clean out afterwards.
- Hold the potty as your child stands up – you don't want the contents all over the floor.

- Always wipe a girl's bottom from front to back, not the other way round.
- Empty the contents of the potty in the loo and wipe it clean.
- Wash your hands and your child's hands.

Nappies or not
Once your child has started using the potty, you have a choice between putting him in pants, in trainer pants (pants made of towelling with a waterproof outer covering), in pull-ups (like disposable nappies, but pants-shaped), or keeping him in nappies. Many parents use a combination, putting their child in pants at home, using trainer pants or pull-ups when they go out, and putting a nappy on for naps or long journeys.

Accidents
Be prepared for accidents, especially with wees. All children have them. Accidents are never convenient and are often annoying, but you'll be helping your child if you can be as sympathetic as possible about them, rather than getting cross. Saying things like, 'Never mind – it doesn't matter' – even if it does – will help him feel better.

Using the loo
When your child eventually progresses to using the loo, it may be less daunting for him at first if you put a toddler seat on it. This makes it a lot easier to sit on, as long as the seat is firm. If you put a low stool or step in front of it, it'll be easier for him to get on to the loo. Boys might prefer sitting down to wee too, at the beginning.

LET'S PRETEND

Some time between two and three your toddler will begin to understand that people have a role — that mummies and daddies behave in certain ways and that babies behave differently, for example. So 'being Mummy' for a while is fun.

Once your toddler begins to understand that different people do different things he can use his improved memory to generate more interesting pretend play, and string together two or three different activities.

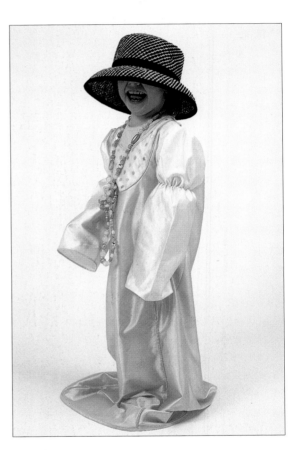

MAKE-BELIEVE PLAY

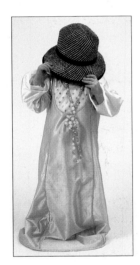

By two-and-a-half most children are at this stage: tucking up their dolls for the night, vacuuming over the vestiges of this morning's breakfast with their push-along toys, or noisily revving the motor in their cardboard box cars. And most of them know instinctively that the best place for this is in the kitchen while you are cooking.

Most of the time he will play on his own, but he will check in with you frequently during the game to reassure himself and to fill you in on the latest happenings, in the unlikely event that you hadn't heard the drone of his monologue. And if you're really good you may even be allocated a bit part along with his soft toys.

By two-and-a-half your toddler may well be able to join in with other children. He has finally realised how to make friends. He is beginning to understand how to relate to people

'Daniel (32 months) is learning to share. He'll give his friends toys and say "You have that one and I'll have this one." He's always giving his baby brother toys, although of course he does take them away again, but he sometimes remembers what I say about giving him another one instead.'

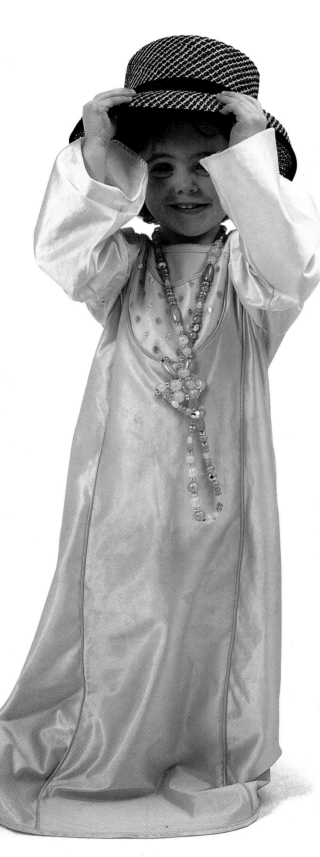

'Susannah (31 months) has worn the same Snow White outfit every day for about three weeks now. I wash it every night and, luckily, it's dry by morning. She absolutely refuses to put anything else on. At least I got good value from that purchase!'

in differing ways and how to co-operate with them. But none of this is very sophisticated yet. At play with a friend your toddler's co-operation usually depends on the shared aim of a particular game, and once the activity is finished, the ability to share may rapidly disappear. Indeed, during the game much of the conversation of toddlers involves either telling each other what to do or, alternatively, asserting what they are doing.

TOYS TO LOOK FOR

Children don't need many props for pretend play – most of the action goes on in their heads, or with everyday objects that just happen to fit the bill. But there are a few things that can help:

- dressing up box – fill it with natty outfits you haven't worn since the 70s or jumble sale finds, particularly hats. Handbags or a small suitcase for trips to Africa/the office/Sainsbury's are also invaluable
- toy people, animals, cars – so that your toddler can make and break his own world, as many times a day as he likes
- dolls and teddies of different sizes are needed to people his games and take the shouts and cuddles without answering back
- scaled-down versions of real domestic tools, or plastic versions of tool kits are good
- a box of face paints – for when he has to be a pirate/tiger/butterfly.

CONCENTRATION

A brief six months makes a marked difference to your toddler's ability to concentrate, to remember, and to use her hands. All these things add up to a toddler whose play is more involved, more detailed and lasts longer than before.

Your child may love to play with a doll's house, because now she is able to stand the figures up, steadying them with her free hand, and invent things for them to do. Or she may be equally fascinated by cars or model dinosaurs, for the same reason.

Toddlers often become obsessed by one particular sort of toy, spending hours each day with their toy farm or their cooking set, endlessly elaborating their games. 'Alex (34 months) is completely obsessed with trains. I think he always was. At first it was just Thomas and then all Thomas's friends and now it's any trains. I think it's his dad's fault really for encouraging him, but I suppose it's quite harmless.'

This new attention to detail is also reflected in the way your toddler looks

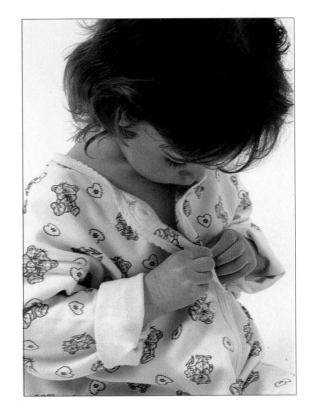

at books or photographs – picking out the tiniest detail. Now she may enjoy books that have something to find on each page. 'Every night for the past week we've read the Apple Tree Farm book where there's a little yellow duck to find on each page. Katherine (30 months) hugs herself with excitement every time she finds the duck before I do. Which just happens to be on almost every page.'

IMAGINATIVE DRAWING

Drawing and painting become easier now because your toddler has learnt how to hold the paper steady with one hand while drawing with the other. Each hand can now have a different job, rather than acting in unison because her hands can now operate on their own. And this frees her to think her wonderful thoughts about what she is drawing today.

'I have noticed a recent change in Rachel's (36 months) drawings. They have much more control and she now holds the pencils or pens between thumb and fingers. Her pictures are no longer scribbled but quite precise and she concentrates quite intensely.'

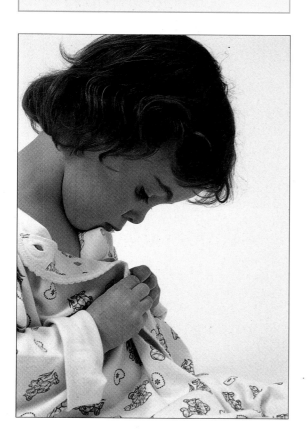

QUIET PLAY

If you have a very active toddler, who is most happy running around the garden in large circles or climbing on the furniture, you may want to find ways of encouraging 'quiet play'. Games with natural materials are good for calming a child and encouraging concentration.

WATER

If you're working in the kitchen, put your toddler in an apron and wellies and stand him on a sturdy chair next to the sink. Put lots of newspaper on the floor and fill the sink with warm water. Give him old plastic bottles or a colander to play with. Plastic tubing and funnels (as used for making home-made beer) are good fun, too, and if he seems to be getting bored, a squeeze of washing-up liquid or a little powder paint to colour the water will start the interest all over again. (Keep the water warm.)

PLAYDOUGH

The simplest way to make playdough is to measure out equal amounts of flour and salt (8oz/225g of each is fine) and slowly add water, mixing as you pour, to make a stiff but pliable dough. You can add food colouring to the water, to colour the dough, or mix powder paint with the flour. Making the dough is fun in itself, but your toddler will also enjoy squeezing it through his fingers, rolling it into a ball and then trying to 'make snakes' by rolling the ball on a flat surface. A rolling pin and pastry cutters are useful and so is a patty-tin, or an empty egg box. He can put a playdough cake into each section and decorate with dried beans or raisins. He can also squeeze the dough through a garlic press and watch it come out as 'worms'.

PHYSICAL SKILLS AT 2½

Your toddler is advancing rapidly, learning new physical and mental skills every day, and is proud of it.

By now your child may be able to walk upstairs confidently, one step at a time. He may even have got the hang of walking downstairs holding on to the banister or wall, although if he's tired or there are things in his way he will revert to sliding down on his bottom. He can run well in a straight line, and can manage corners without having to fling his arms out for balance. He can also climb small slides and climbing frames and will probably enjoy walking along the top of a low wall, holding your hand for reassurance.

If he's not your first child, your toddler may well be more advanced in his physical skills than his brother or sister was at this age. This is because he's learnt a lot from watching them at play. 'I used to think that Charlotte, Ben's older sister, fell over the football every time she ran up to it because we didn't get out of the flat to play often, but Ben is amazingly proficient, and yet we still don't get to the park as often as I'd like. But I suppose he does have Charlotte to teach him to play while I'm busy and they make up all sorts of ball games between them.'

He may be able to push and pull large wheeled toys pretty

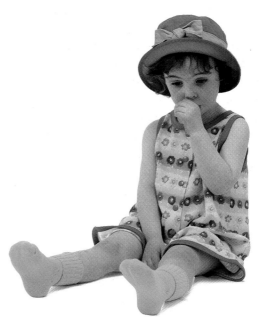

skilfully, although any obstructions like brothers and sisters lying in his chosen path will frustrate him because steering round things is still hard. He can walk on tip-toe, if you show him how, and be as tall as a giraffe or maybe even as tall as daddy. Some toddlers, especially those with parents who have time to practise with them, can throw a ball (if a little stiffly) and kick a football without falling over, although it probably won't go far or in the expected direction.

ROUGH AND TUMBLE PLAY

Some toddlers love rough and tumble play and others steer well clear. Some parents have equally clear-cut views – either feeling that it's fun or that it encourages aggression. If your toddler is keen, he'll rough and tumble with his friends at any opportunity, running, laughing and wrestling in turns, and he'll quickly learn which friends like to do the same. Toddlers seem to know instinctively whether it's right for them so let your child take the lead. After all, there's no evidence that rough and tumble play leads on to real fights whereas your toddler does become fitter when he plays vigorously, and a bout of rough and tumble is certainly vigorous. But even more importantly, spontaneous rough and tumble play is just fun.

'One of Katy's (35 months) favourite games at the moment is wrestling on the bed. Whenever she and her daddy are upstairs, there's a lot of giggling and tickling that goes on. I'm not sure who comes down looking more flushed and excited!'

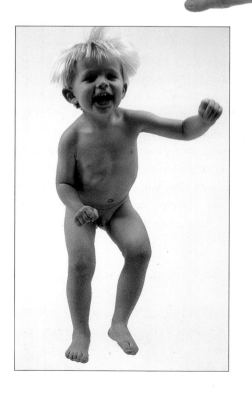

'Elizabeth (32 months) tried a lot of new things at gym-tots today, but she took one look at the big ladder and said "I'll leave that for when I'm a little bit older, Mummy." I think the height scared her, because she was actually very confident on most of the other equipment.'

Physically, your toddler has made enormous progress. Standing on one leg requires phenomenal balance, strength and co-ordination at this age

STARTING AT PLAYGROUP

Between the ages of two and three, your child is likely to blossom in both stature and confidence. Introducing her to a playgroup at this stage can meet any needs that she has to forge ahead in a safe place with a degree of independence.

Playgroups, or pre-schools, are now available for most under-fives. They are run by trained workers with the help of volunteer parents on a rota basis. Playgroups offer children the opportunity to learn through play,

'To my relief Chloe is beginning to develop the ability to assert herself. She will say "Don't push me", or "I'm playing with that", or just "No". Very loudly but not aggressively. The other day she said "It's not nice to hit people," to another child. It proves the things you say do make an impression.'

with a variety of activities including painting, playdough, water or sand play, puzzles, construction toys, and a dressing-up corner.

Very often, starting at playgroup is the child's first time away from her mother and this transition can be a big step, which children deal with in a variety of ways. Some will head off into the bustle of the play area, scarcely glancing back, leaving their parent feeling slightly bemused and surplus to requirements. Others will

play happily, apparently oblivious to your presence until you move towards the door, at which point you become vital to them. Many children cling tightly to their parent's hand, wanting to get to the play area, but scared to leave you in case you disappear.

In order for your child to be left there happily, it is important that you both enjoy the ambience of the chosen playgroup. She will pick up on any misgivings that you may have, so take time to find the right place for both of you. You can always visit playgroups before you commit yourself to one, and it might be useful to look out for the following features:

• greetings and a warm welcome from the staff, particularly for your child

• a bright, friendly atmosphere, with plenty of the children's pictures covering the walls of the premises

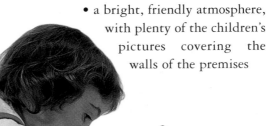

- a scrupulously clean environment
- child-size toilets, or steps to help children to reach the loos
- a recognised security routine for collecting children after each session
- a safe environment, where children cannot leave supervised areas without an adult
- an interest table, where children can bring in objects from home
- access to a play area outside.

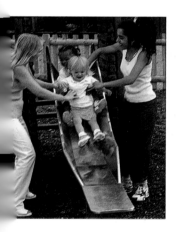

GETTING OFF TO A GOOD START

Your child may be very excited at the prospect of playgroup, but a little more hesitant when she arrives there. For the first two sessions, try to make sure you are available to stay if you need to. You may find that staying for the first session is enough, and you can leave after she has settled into the second session. When you do leave her, let her know that you are going, and that you will collect her when it is finished. If she cries, her tears will probably be over more quickly if you give her a quick hug and kiss and then leave, allowing one of the workers to divert her attention. Very often children cry because they don't like the reality of separation, but they usually settle down soon after it has taken place.

If your child cries every day for a number of weeks, you may be expecting too much of her. If she is not yet three, she may benefit from waiting another term. If she is going every day, try cutting it down to every other day and see if that makes her feel more relaxed. The staff at the playgroup will be happy to talk to you about how she is settling in.

PLAYGROUPS...

- are run by a combination of trained workers and parent volunteers
- are encouraged to have a ratio of one adult to every five children
- generally cost between £2 and £4 per session
- have sessions that last about two-and-a-half hours, morning or afternoon
- normally offer two sessions a week to start with, and build up to more as your child's confidence grows
- expect your child to be out of nappies during the day.

A typical playgroup session may run like this:
- arrive at playgroup, hang up coat on child's own named peg
- free play
- group together for songs, milk and biscuits, talk about the weather and the day of the week
- trip to the toilet for everyone
- more free play in small groups
- group together for children's news, looking at interest table, and story time
- parents collect children.

You can make playgroup simple by:
- dressing your child in clothes that she can easily remove for visits to the loo
- dressing your child in clothes that can get paint or playdough on them
- dropping her off on time
- more importantly, collect her in good time
- being prepared for tiredness (and therefore grumpiness), for the first few weeks
- inviting a friend home for her to play with, either for lunch or later on if she's tired. She'll look forward to playgroup days even more with a familiar friendly face.

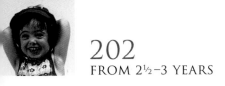
THE NEXT BABY

If you or your partner is pregnant for the second time, you're probably finding it a different kind of experience from the first time around.

For many parents, a second pregnancy isn't as exciting and absorbing as the first. You have your first child to look after and you may find that you have less time to think about the coming baby. Many mothers also feel much more tired during second pregnancies. You'll probably have different worries, too. Many parents expecting their second child wonder how on earth they'll manage to cope with the demands of a new baby as well as the demands of their older child. They may also feel sad at the loss of the one-to-one relationship that they currently have with their first child and wonder if they'll ever be able to love another child as much.

Many parents expecting a second baby find themselves torn between wanting the baby and not wanting their first child to be upset by the new arrival. As Kate put it: 'I really want Jamie to have a brother or sister, but I feel really guilty about turning his little world upside down. It feels like I'm betraying him.'

Although parents worry about their child being jealous when a new brother or sister is born, it's quite normal for the child to feel that way. It would actually be more surprising if he didn't. You're unlikely to be able to prevent your child feeling any jealousy at all, but you may be able to take some steps to help minimise these painful feelings.

In particular, try if you can to avoid any other major changes in your child's routine – such as moving from a cot to a bed or starting using the potty or beginning playgroup – around the time a new baby is expected. Having his special place as the baby snatched from him is about as much change as he can cope with right now.

Before the baby arrives:
• Let your child spend time with other children who have babies in their families, if you can.
• Talk to him about what babies are like and what they can do. Don't tell him that the baby will be someone he can play with – she won't be at the beginning.
• Show him photographs of himself as a baby.
• Show him where the baby is and let him feel.
• Sing songs together to the baby.
• Read stories about children whose mothers have a baby.
• Some children like to have a doll or teddy as their 'baby'.

SAYING HELLO TO THE NEW BABY

Like Sarah, some parents are careful to arrange their child's first meeting with their new brother or sister so that they can give their full attention to the child: 'When Amy came to see me after Holly was born, I made sure that I hadn't got Holly in my arms so that I could give Amy a hug.'

Many parents, like Amanda, get a present to give to their child from the new baby: 'Luke was far more interested in the tricycle that was a present from his new baby sister than he was in the sister.'

AFTER THE BABY IS BORN

Try to:
• Involve your child in looking after the baby, if he wants to, but don't insist.
• Talk to him about what the baby is doing.
• Ask his opinion about what the baby wants.
• Point out things he can do that the baby can't, but try and avoid giving the impression that the baby is silly or that he is 'better' than the baby.
• When you have to give your attention to the baby – when you're feeding her or bathing her, for example – make sure that your child has plenty of toys to amuse himself with, or read or sing or talk to him.
• Find time to do things with your child without the baby, if you can – these can be ordinary things like reading him a story or bathing him, or special things like outings.
• Arrange things so that your child gets attention from both his parents rather than mainly from his father while his mother looks after the baby.
• Keep to his routine as much as you can.

TRY NOT TO:
• always make him wait until you've finished with the baby – make the baby wait sometimes
• use the baby as an excuse for not being able to attend to him
• be over-protective of the baby – let him handle the baby and if he seems too rough, explain that the baby is tiny and needs to be handled gently
• make an issue of it if he reverts to babyish behaviour and tell him he's much too big for that now – just go with it and it will pass
• make negative comparisons between him and the baby.

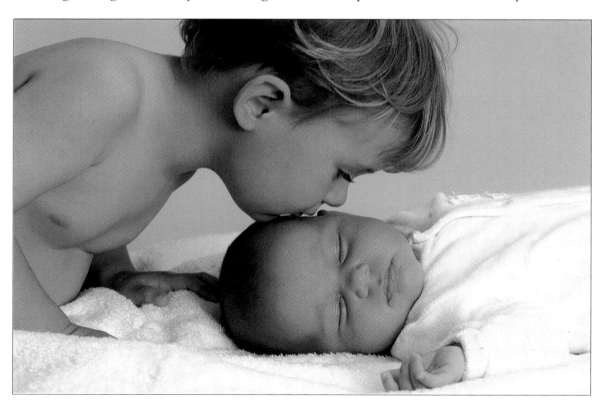

YOUR BABY –
THREE PLUS

Your three-year-old is probably a lot easier to live with now. Three things have helped: she's more competent, more realistic, and she has begun to use words as well as actions to express her feelings.

Your three-year-old's new competence comes from her increased mastery over her body. These days she needs you less to take care of her, and more to help her to get on with what she wants to do. A peg by the door for her coat, means she can hang it up for herself, and a plate of sandwiches handed to her means she can carry them to the table herself. Naturally, tantrums don't disappear overnight but there are usually fewer than before. 'When Isaac (37 months) has a tantrum, it's usually because I haven't done something right. This morning after two attempts to draw Eeyore himself he asked me to. I drew him from a side view but with only one eye – a complete disaster!'

Your three-year-old's realism is based on her increasingly sophisticated awareness of what it means for you and she to be two separate people – an idea that she's been developing for the last couple of years. Now, at last, she begins to treat you as a thinking, feeling, loving person, just

like her. If she can't manage to get in the car without dropping her ice lolly it is no longer necessarily your fault, although she may still cry with frustration. If you curse when you slam the front door and realise at that precise moment that the keys are still on the table inside she will give you a hug to make it better. And perhaps most important of all for an easier life, she can now more easily wait her turn, because she knows that other people get sad just like she does when they don't have a go (though you'd be hoping for too much if you always expected her to wait in line peaceably).

Your three-year-old is ready to broaden her horizons – to begin to look out from you, your partner and her siblings towards other children. She will use the experience of her first relationship with you as a model on which to make future relationships. Many of her relationships will be easily made and quickly forgotten – some may only last the length of a

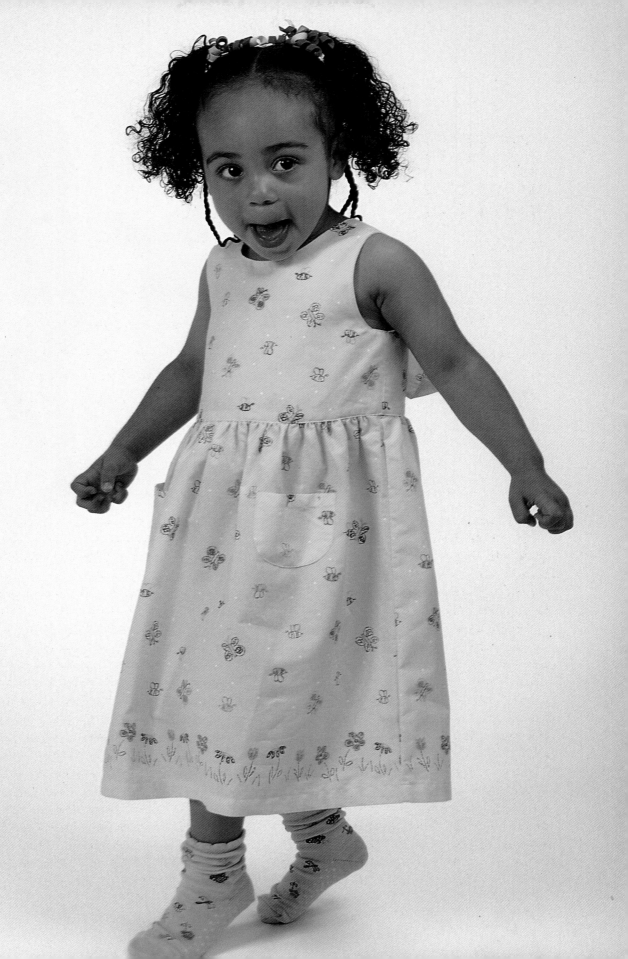

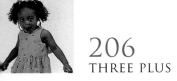

visit to the doctor's surgery, or a one-off session at a toddler group. But reaching out or at least watching closely is the order of the day. By three, your child has learnt to treat people differently from each other. 'I've noticed that Thomas (41 months) is quite punchy and kicky with his brother and sister, but seems to know this is not acceptable in other situations.'

Three-year-olds often become more affectionate and confiding than before. Hugging you when it strikes them afresh that they love you, rather than because they want a cuddle themselves and whispering of things that they know shouldn't be spoken aloud: 'That lady's got green hair, mummy', or of their special secrets: 'I've got a sheep in my pocket'. Your three-year-old may also be noticeably more affectionate than before to siblings (particularly younger ones). In some families affection and consolation may be sought from someone other

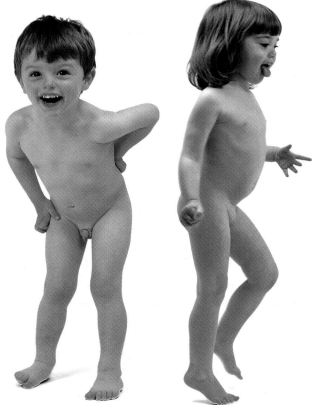

than mum or dad, if that person is familiar. 'The other day Jess (39 months) hurt herself and came running in crying but she didn't quite know who to go to because Angela, who we see every day, and I were sitting next to each other on the sofa.'

Most three-year-olds want to get 'it' right, and to please you, and are happy when they do. So this is a good time to start using all that competence and dawning realism to good effect in the real world, as well as in the world of toys. 'When we go to Sainsbury's, Helen (39 months) has her own list with pictures of the things she wants to buy – it's usually all fruit, because I can't draw much else – but she's really proud of herself, reminding me what we need, and saying 'silly mummy' when I draw red apples and they only have Cox's and Granny Smiths in.' Show her how to use her sorting skills to help lay the table, or to tidy away her toys. Use her skill in

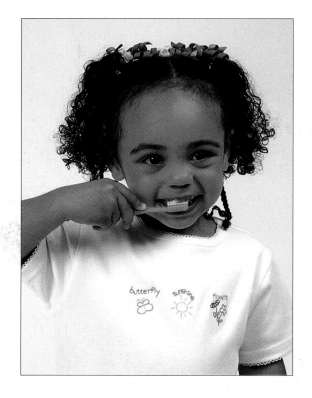

adapting to people to help keep your baby amused. All these activities can be a shared pleasure, and a pleasure which with sensitive handling can become an everyday part of your child's sense of herself – someone who can help, and is proud and happy to do so.

QUESTIONS

Her questions, as ever, are indications of what she is thinking. Right now the wonders of 'what?' 'where?', 'who?' and 'why?' are uppermost in her mind. She has moved on from simply wanting to know the names of things to asking what makes them work. She is asking about things that are hidden – emotions and physical forces as well as the past and the future.

A three-year-old may even talk about things that happened a long time ago. 'Yesterday we were watching Teletubbies and when Callum (38 months) saw a seal he said, "we saw a seal by the water with the big wheel." I was amazed because he was remembering a holiday we'd been on ten months before, and yet neither Duncan nor I had talked to him about it.'

By the age of three, most children can understand the idea of feelings and you can help her find words for her feelings in a matter-of-fact way. For example, 'I know it makes you angry when you have to go to bed, but you'll get very tired if you don't', or 'You're sad because you won't see Daddy again until next week, but he'll be thinking about you'. It also helps if you can talk about your own feelings in the same way. Children can learn to name their emotions in the same way that they learn the colours.

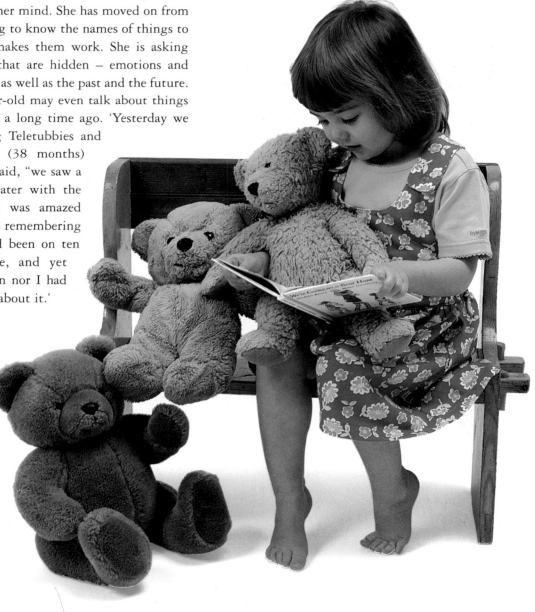

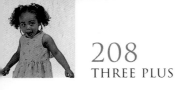
DIARY OF A THREE-YEAR-OLD

Jake is three. He has a baby brother, Matthew, who is four months old. His mother, Caroline, doesn't work outside the home. Dale, his father, is out at work during the day.

7am

Jake wakes up and gets out of bed. He takes his night-time nappy off and goes to the loo. Then he dresses himself in the clothes that Caroline has put out for him the previous night. He is usually quite happy to wear what Caroline has chosen for him, though sometimes he decides he wants to wear something else, and empties the contents of his cupboard until he finds what he wants. He then plays by himself in his bedroom.

8am

While Caroline is feeding Matthew, Dale gets up and takes Jake downstairs for breakfast.

8.45am

Dale leaves for work. On three mornings a week, Jake goes to pre-school, and Dale takes him on his way to work. On mornings when he's at home, he plays with his toys or watches cartoons on television while Caroline has her breakfast. Caroline used not to let him watch cartoons, but she's now relented and allows him 30–45 minutes a day.

9am

On Mondays, Caroline takes Jake to a playgroup in a village a few miles from where she lives. She goes there rather than to a local one

because she meets up with her friend, Nicki, whom she met at her NCT antenatal class, and Nicki's daughter, Yasmin. Jake and Yasmin are great friends and love playing together.

If Jake isn't going to pre-school or playgroup, Caroline, Jake and Matthew usually go shopping. Jake likes to know exactly how many shops they're going to go in before he'll be able to go and play in the ball pool in the shopping centre's play area. 'He likes everything planned,' says Caroline. 'Every morning, he says "What are we going to do today, Mummy?" It's important to him to know what's going to be happening.'

12.30pm

Lunchtime. Jake's favourite is a picnic lunch with sandwiches and fruit, though Caroline usually gives him a cooked lunch and keeps the picnic for an afternoon snack.

1pm

Jake has a nap for a couple of hours. Before he goes to sleep, he insists on having a drink and a story. 'His little routines are very important to him,' Caroline says.

3pm

Jake wakes up from his nap. If the weather is fine, Caroline, Jake and Matthew usually go

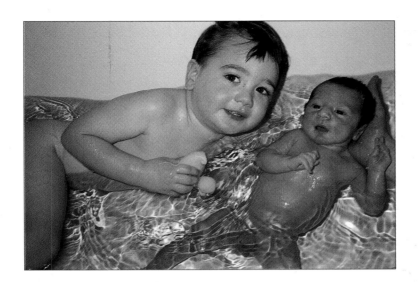

to the park. Jake likes to ride there on his bike, which he's very proud of. They usually meet up with friends in the park. Jake likes to play football, and to climb on the rope climbing frame, which Caroline thinks is alarmingly high. 'It used to freak me, but you have to let him go for it.'

When the weather isn't so good, Jake stays at home and plays with his toys. He prefers Caroline to choose for him what he's going to play with. He likes painting and sticking, and particularly enjoys making cards with his ink stamps. He also likes construction toys, and to play pretend games with his doctor's kit or his tea set. 'He likes to make tea for me,' says Caroline. Sometimes they make cakes. Jake likes to make Rice Krispie cakes, which he knows how to do by himself.

5pm

Jake plays by himself while Caroline gets his tea ready, then has his tea.

5.45pm

Bathtime. Caroline tries to make sure that she starts getting Jake ready for bed before he becomes too tired, otherwise bedtime can

become difficult. Jake and Matthew go in the bath together and Jake helps Caroline to bath Matthew. Caroline takes Matthew out of the bath and adds some hotter water and bubbles for Jake. After his bath, Jake puts his bath toys away and gets into his pyjamas.

Once he's in his pyjamas, Jake stays upstairs, preparing for bed. He plays in his room, or he helps Caroline to dress Matthew, or he chooses some books for bedtime reading.

6.30pm

Dale will usually have come home while Jake is in the bath. He reads to Jake and Matthew while Caroline gets supper ready. Jake likes to sit up in bed so that he can see the pictures in the book. He makes sure there's room for Matthew on the bed and explains to Matthew what's happening in the story.

7pm

Lights out. Jake is happy to go to sleep on his own, but he likes to have his bedroom door open so that he can hear where his parents are. Once he's gone to sleep, he now rarely wakes until the morning.

Caroline has found that life with Jake has got easier in the last six months. 'He understands more, so you can reason with him more,' she says. 'And you can hold a real conversation with him now.' She's also found that she needs to be more consistent in what she says to him. 'He remembers what you say to him and notices if you give a different explanation from one you've given before or that someone else has given. He's really quite a challenge to be with!'

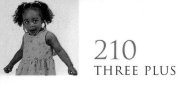

PLAY AT THREE YEARS

Your three-year-old's increasing ability to make believe, to share and to empathise make him a much better companion for other children. His heightened awareness that others also have feelings allows him to begin to empathise when a playmate wants the toy he is using or clamours to have first go.

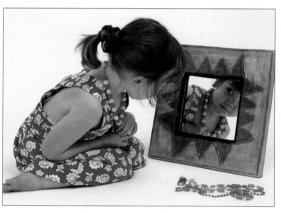

props. Your three-year-old may people his games in his imagination, or with one or two soft toys, so he may not need you to join in as much, yet you are still his major inspiration. Many young children play make-believe games where the mother

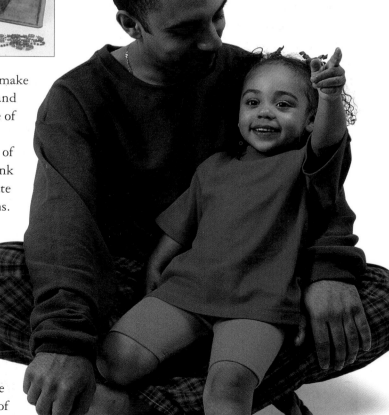

Empathy and a longer memory make sharing toys and attention, and taking turns, all possible (at least some of the time).

Many three-year-olds spend most of their day being somebody else. 'I think Robert (40 months) has been a pirate every day now for the last three months. To be honest it's wearing a bit thin, and if I have to tie one more pirate's scarf I'll scream, but he won't answer if we don't call him Pirate Jake.' Now he's more insightful his role plays are less stereotypical and more inventive and because the drama is unfolding in his head he will be able to act things out with the minimum of

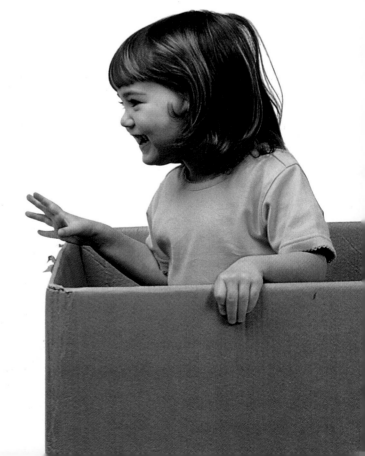

PICTURE THIS

Drawing at this age is still largely for the sheer fun of using pencils and paints to make a mark. It's best not to ask most three-year-olds what they have drawn as they will probably either be baffled or feel that they have somehow failed. Children's ability to draw certain shapes follows a pattern – circles first, then vertical lines and then horizontal lines. Yet, occasionally a three-year-old is ready to draw a circle, with or without some squiggles inside it and label it as 'mummy' or 'me'. It will be months or even years before he will draw in legs, arms and a body in that order.

'Callum (39 months) has been painting animals at playgroup, and he tells me what they are but it's hard to see, so I do ask where all the different bits are.'

'When Eleanor (40 months) draws a body she joins all the bits together with squiggles, but her brother Scott, at the same age drew all the bits disjointed.'

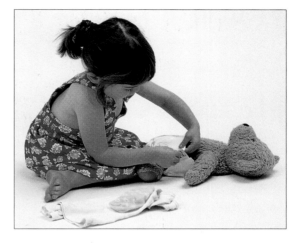

berates her child to 'watch out', 'hurry up', 'stop being silly', and so on. Your three-year-old is learning from you what to say to himself. He probably also has your relationship with your partner taped, and if you watch carefully you can see him copying your looks and attitudes here too. Nothing is private when there are small children around.

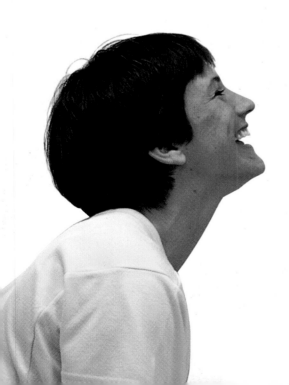

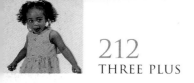

YOUR THREE-YEAR-OLD'S SKILLS

Your three-year-old is learning to master his body, and loving every minute of it – walking with a longer step, forwards, backwards or sideways, and running with confidence, around obstacles as well as in a straight line.

Young children love to test their growing physical ability, and to invent as many variations on the basic skills as possible. These days when she pushes or pulls large toys it's not to help her balance but to squeeze every ounce of fun out of walking. Dancing is a new-found ability that adds excitement to the skill of walking on tiptoe.

'Rebecca (36 months) loves dancing. Yesterday she did two gallops and then three claps, two gallops and three claps over and over again. Quite rhythmic really.'

Many children of this age love jumping, and may be able to get 30cm off the ground, while others spend more time climbing than on the floor.

A rule of thumb is that if he thinks he can do it – he probably can. Calls of 'be careful' are likely to undermine his faith in himself, just as quickly as being pushed beyond his powers.

And pedalling a car or bike turns that boring trip to the shops or to and from playgroup into something much more adventurous. 'Nick (44 months) loves riding his bicycle with the stabilisers on, pedalling furiously and trying to keep up with his older brother and sister.'

LANGUAGE

For the next couple of years your child will want to talk almost all the time. She may only know 500 words right now but it seems as though she wants to try them in every possible combination and at every possible volume. Most three-year-olds are one-person acts – whispering, shouting and talking high or low to get their point across. She'll be able to tell you her full name, her age and maybe even her address.

Familiarity and ritual are comforting to young children, which is why many of them demand favourite stories over and over, repeatedly count to ten by heart, and tunelessly chant 'the alphabet song'. Yet most three-year-olds don't appreciate the actual meaning of numbers beyond two or three, or recognise written letters. Even the names of the colours are just so

IMITATING HERSELF

While learning to thread beads many three-year-olds stick out their tongue with concentration and in imitation of the thread passing through the eye of the bead – an imitative trick that they may first have learnt when they were only a few hours old (see page 10).

The same sort of thing happens when your child first cuts with scissors. Concentrating hard, your child may open the scissors and her mouth wide at the same time, and then close them both together as well. This sort of unintentional imitation helps her to get to grips with this new way of using her hands.

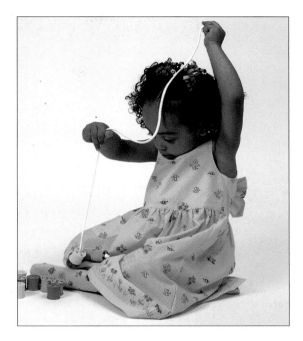

many words, with the average three-year-old matching only two or three of them. Many three-year-olds still have immature pronunciation, using sounds made at the front of the mouth to substitute for those made in the middle. 'Isaac (37 months) can't pronounce "c" at the beginning of words. I love it when he asks me for a "tiss and a tuddle".'

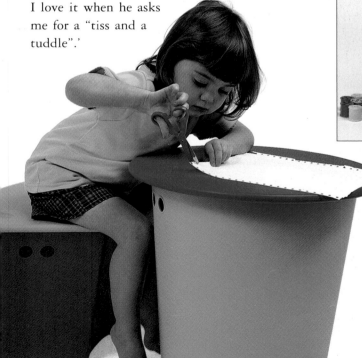

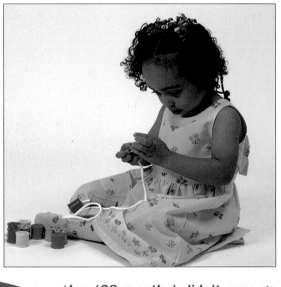

'Joe (38 months) didn't ever go to a crèche but Charlie, his brother, did and they have completely different accents and vocabularies. I think Charlie's language is a lot more childlike because he's been with children all the time.'

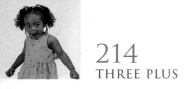

SLEEP FOR THREE-YEAR-OLDS

Sleep patterns are by now quite firmly entrenched, and most children are able to sleep for up to 12 hours a night. However, many still do not return to sleep unless they have woken you up.

It's never too late to start a bedtime routine. With a routine, everyone knows what is expected. However, your child may still decide that she isn't tired just yet. By giving them time and letting them finish what they are doing (within reason), they may feel more in control of the process and amenable to your wishes.

YOUR CHILD'S BEDROOM

This should be somewhere that he enjoys going to, and will play in happily. Make going to the bedroom a pleasure by having books and pictures to look at and toys to play with in there. The end of the day should also be a time

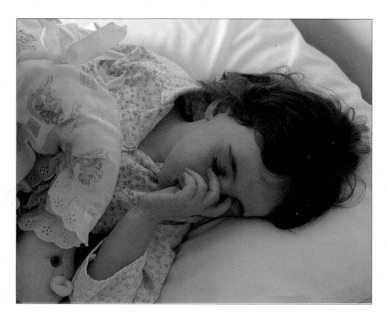

to be together, talking and reading stories. It's likely that you will be apart for some of the day by now, whether you are back at work, or he is at nursery or playgroup, so there will be lots to catch up on. Although you may be tired, an extra half hour spent talking to your child can pay dividends. This is a good time to allow him to express any worries, and to reassure him before sleep. Try to ensure that you leave enough time for this, and take your child's fears seriously, as this age often brings with it new worries.

The world of the child can be a scary place at times, populated as it is by giants and monsters. You may find that on occasion he has nightmares or, much more rarely, night terrors.

NIGHTMARES

A nightmare is a bad dream, from which your child may awake, crying and frightened. They take place during the dreaming phase of sleep, that is, during a light sleeping period. He will need reassurance and cuddling, but should soon return to sleep. It isn't always possible to find the cause of a nightmare, but by talking to your child about it, you can put it in perspective and tell him that it was not real. Although most nightmares will have no root cause, if you find that your child is waking regularly with bad dreams, you could try to find out if there is anything causing him anxiety.

NIGHT TERRORS

Night terrors take place when the body is in a deep sleeping phase, that is, not in the usual dreaming state. They tend to be announced by the child screaming, and when you get there, he is likely to be wide-eyed and looking petrified. At the time, he will be inconsolable, however, he will have no recollection of this in the morning, and although he seems to be awake, he is unconscious of his behaviour. Try not to wake him, and he should settle back into sleep, unless he is in danger of hurting himself. Luckily, these night terrors are very rare, affecting only about 3% of children, and fortunately, they are more terrifying for the parents, as the children will have forgotten all about them by the next day.

MAKING BEDTIME APPEALING

By the time your child is three, he will probably be in his own bed. If you don't want him to get out of bed at night, try the following:
• Be consistent. If he keeps coming down, keep taking him back.
• Let him keep a light on, and a cassette player with a tape close by, so he has some distraction.
• Reward him for staying in bed – but don't get tied into buying presents every day.
• If he uses any sort of comforter, let him continue using it until he is settled into his night-time routine.
• Potter close to his room for a little while. He will be aware of your presence, which will help him to settle into sleep.
• Make sure your child knows that if he needs you, you will come to him.

DRY AT NIGHT

One of the first steps towards becoming dry at night is staying dry during a nap. If this is happening often, try leaving your child's nappy off during naps.

If he's regularly waking in the morning with a dry nappy, you can take the next step of letting him sleep at night without a nappy. Put a waterproof cover over the mattress to protect it against the inevitable accidents. Some parents put their children to bed without pyjama bottoms or pants when they first sleep without nappies, to minimise washing.

Make sure your child uses the potty or goes to the loo last thing at night. Leave a potty beside his bed for him to use if he needs it in the night and switch on a low light of some kind so that he can see what he's doing.

Another strategy is to 'lift' your child when you go to bed yourself, taking him out of bed and sitting him on the potty or loo to encourage a wee.

If your child is regularly wetting the bed, you may need to put him back in nappies and wait until he's consistently waking with his nappy dry again. It may help his self-esteem if you present this as being a

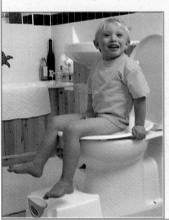

way of giving him a good night's sleep for a while, which is better than the disturbed nights he's been getting with wet beds.

CARING FOR YOUR SICK CHILD

When a child becomes ill, parents are naturally worried. Even a mild temperature can cause a child to be listless and sleepy and it becomes quite obvious, even to a new parent, that their child is not well. These days you are often on your own or with a partner who is as inexperienced as you are, so dealing with a sick child can be frightening. Here are some guidelines to help you cope.

Start by taking your child's temperature. If you or other people with whom the child has been in contact have been ill with a cold or virus then the child probably has the same thing. Colds, sore throats, ear infections, and tummy bugs all usually have short incubation periods of just a few days (the time between catching the illness and the signs appearing). The childhood fevers such as chickenpox often have longer incubation periods and these are all listed in the A–Z of health later in the book. Urine or kidney infections (also called cystitis) are not usually passed from one person to another but will still cause a raised temperature.

HOW TO TAKE YOUR CHILD'S TEMPERATURE

Check your child's temperature with a mercury thermometer, a fever strip or an ear thermometer. Ear thermometers are relatively expensive and although they do give a very quick and accurate reading it is worthwhile learning to read a mercury thermometer. These are available from any pharmacist.

First of all shake the mercury down towards the bulb. Hold the thermometer at the end opposite the bulb and shake down. To read the thermometer you will need to rotate it slightly and look for the level of the mercury. Practise

this, and if you have any problems ask your health visitor to show you. You will need to keep shaking it down until the mercury is at 35°C or less. Now place the bulb end under the armpit and cuddle your child towards you, keeping the thermometer in place for two minutes. Then read it again. Don't forget to shake it down each time you use it. Avoid putting a mercury thermometer in a child's mouth to read temperature in case the child accidentally bites it.

These days doctors and nurses use the Centigrade scale and the cut off point is usually taken as 37°C. If you decide to buy an ear thermometer follow the instructions included in the pack. You may find that the normal temperature range given is slightly different from conventional mercury thermometers. A normal temperature is always reassuring but if the child still doesn't seem right, check it again in a little while. The normal pattern with many viral illnesses is for the temperature to fluctuate up and down for the first day or two of the illness prior to more specific symptoms developing.

TREATING A FEVER

The aim of treatment of a fever is to keep the temperature as normal as possible during this period. This is done with paracetamol (syrup or dissolving tablets or, in cases of severe vomiting, paracetamol suppositories inserted into the back passage).

Paracetamol treatment is accompanied by tepid sponging. To do this remove all of the child's clothing except the nappy. Take a bowl of lukewarm water and sponge the child all over. The water should evaporate on the skin so don't dry with a towel. If the temperature is very high you can speed up the evaporation by fanning with an electric fan or even using a newspaper. Be warned that your child will not like it! However it is very important that you do this continuously until you succeed in lowering the temperature. In an acute feverish illness you will find that the temperature will start to go up again within a few hours and you start the process all over again. You might prefer to try a lukewarm bath which can be just as effective but again your child is unlikely to enjoy it. Nevertheless these measures are essential to bring a temperature down where paracetamol on its own has not been effective.

WHEN TO CALL A DOCTOR

Be aware of the following signs that your baby may be ill:
- off feeds (less than half of normal in last 24 hours)
- persistent vomiting
- fast breathing rate, especially if the breathing is noisy and the breathing difficulty has come on suddenly ➤

PARACETAMOL

- **Follow the instructions on the bottle**
Give paracetamol in the dose recommended for the age of the child.
- **Never run out of paracetamol**
Children often become ill at night so make sure your medicine cabinet is stocked up.
- **Repeat the dose**
Paracetamol will last at best for six hours but usually for three or four. However, don't exceed the recommended dose for a 24-hour period as instructed on the bottle.
- **Never wait for a doctor to come before giving paracetamol**
Children may well seem normal an hour after a dose of paracetamol even when they were quite unwell before. This is often why they seem better as soon as the doctor arrives! However, doctors want to assess the illness, not the fever and it can often be easier for a doctor to assess a child who has had paracetamol.
- **Don't give aspirin to the under 12s**
Paracetamol is safer.

- **Give plenty of fluids**
If you have ever had a fever yourself you will know that it upsets your appetite. We can all cope for a few days, even young children, without our normal food intake. We cannot cope without water, however, and a fever means that we lose even more by sweating. So drinks in any form will do. You may need to be patient with young children as they may not want to drink but you must keep trying even if this means patiently giving the drinks from a spoon. Avoid high sugar drinks with tummy bugs.
- **Be prepared to nurse your child during the night if need be**
The temperature will fluctuate up and down. If there are two of you take it in turns. If you are on your own try to get a relative to help during the day. Nursing a sick child can be exhausting.
- **Avoid wrapping the child up in blankets**
Keep the room reasonably cool and the child in light clothing. Blankets or a duvet could make the temperature worse.

• less than four wet nappies in the last 24 hours
• if the child is sleepy at a time of day when he is normally alert
• irritability
• blood in the bowel motions or in the urine
• a persistently unusual cry
• listlessness or floppiness
• the child is very pale
• delirium – if the temperature is very high the child may seem to be in a sort of a trance and even see things which aren't there (hallucinations)
• skin rash.

Many of these symptoms will result simply from a fever and so you should treat the child's fever immediately. Fever is often the first sign that an illness has begun but it can be 24–28 hours before the signs appear which enable a doctor to make a diagnosis. This is why doctors often do not give antibiotics at the start of an illness even when a child seems quite ill. Once your doctor knows what is causing the fever, and if it is something which responds to antibiotics, then it is safe to treat.

Don't forget that you can call your doctor or nurse if you are really worried. If you do, be prepared to give as much information as possible. Your doctor could well have a list of calls to make to sick patients and it is vital that he or she has enough information to make a decision on who needs to be seen first. Even in an emergency, try to make sure that the person phoning has some information on how serious the case is.

GIVING MEDICINE TO YOUR CHILD

Once you or your doctor have decided that your child needs to have medicine it is important that your child takes it. Many children don't like medicine even though pharmaceutical companies try to make children's medicines taste as nice as possible. If you find that your child does not like paracetamol syrup try every brand and if all else fails buy dissolving tablets and dissolve them in a small amount of her favourite drink.

Special syringes are available to make it easier to measure and administer medicine to babies and children. With one hand cuddle your child towards your chest and with the other place the end of the syringe in the child's mouth. Wait until your child opens her mouth and tip the medicine on to her tongue or down the side of her mouth between her cheek and her gum. You may need to tip her chin up slightly with the same hand to make sure that she doesn't spit it out.

EYE AND EAR DROPS

If your child has conjunctivitis you will need to administer eye drops or ointment. Children do not like having drops put in their eyes so you will need to have patience! It is easier if there is another adult to help you. One adult can cuddle the child keeping her arms by her side while the other gently turns the lower eyelid down and squeezes either the drops or ointment on the inside of the lower eyelid. It is easier than it sounds because it only takes a tiny amount of the drops to dissolve in the tears to enable the drop to spread all over the eyeball. It may seem that most of the dose has come out again especially when the child blinks but don't worry about this. It is trickier if you are on your own and I have in the past resorted to giving drops to a child who is asleep!

Ear drops are fairly straightforward and do not usually cause discomfort. Again if you give your child a firm cuddle keeping the arms in with one arm you will find it easy to give the drops with the other hand.

COPING WITH ACCIDENTS

This section attempts to cover simple emergency procedures in a quick and easy format. However, it is no substitute for real training, so if you have any doubts you should attend an accredited first aid course. Never hesitate to dial 999 if you think it is necessary.

BEE AND WASP STINGS

A wasp sting will not usually be left behind in the skin whereas a bee sting will. The area will be red and swollen. The sting is usually painful for a few minutes so children will invariably be very upset.

Action plan...
• Remove the bee sting with tweezers or by gently scraping with a (blunt!) knife.
• Apply some baking soda (sodium bicarbonate) powder made up with a little water. For wasp stings use vinegar.
• If there is swelling, children over the age of two can be given antihistamines.

Contact the doctor if...
• the child has had a previous severe reaction to a sting
• the child is stung in the mouth
• the child later develops a temperature and the sting area is red, swollen and tender (this can mean the area has become infected)
• if the child becomes breathless or there are other signs of allergy such as a blotchy rash
One or two stings are rarely serious unless the child is known to be allergic to bees or wasps. If there are multiple stings contact a doctor for advice.
➤ ALLERGIES

Dog or other animal bites

Always contact your surgery or hospital for bites that break or tear the skin and if there are cuts/lacerations which may need stitching. Where the skin has not been broken or it is punctured by a tooth you can deal with it yourself. Wash the area carefully and apply an Elastoplast. A tetanus immunisation will only be required if a child has not had their baby immunisations at 8, 12 and 16 weeks. All children are offered a pre-school booster which contains tetanus immunisation. This covers them for a further ten years. Keep an eye on bite areas for a day or two to check for infection – redness, swelling and tenderness.

Seek medical advice immediately for snake bites.

BLEEDING

Action plan...
• With cuts and other injuries which cause bleeding there are two words to remember – pressure and elevation.
• You can stop virtually any bleeding by raising the affected part of the body (above the level of the heart, if possible) and applying pressure with a pad made out of cloth – a piece of clothing or a tea towel.
• In any case of severe bleeding or haemorrhage keep pressing firmly on the bleeding area if

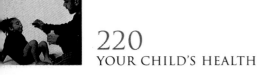
necessary until you can get help from a doctor or ambulance staff.

Small cuts and grazes

Thoroughly clean the wound and apply a dressing such as Elastoplast. Continue to apply some pressure to stop the bleeding as long as there is no glass in the cut. The face, scalp and hands have a very good blood supply so you may need to apply pressure for 15 minutes or more.

Larger cuts

If you think the wound will need stitching take the child to your nearest casualty department or, in the case of rural areas, to your doctor's surgery. Casualty staff may use stitches, steristrips (paper stitches) or surgical glue, but may avoid stitching fingers if they think the injury will continue to swell whereupon the stitches would hamper the blood supply. In cases where a sharp object has punctured the skin don't attempt to remove it. This will be done in hospital where severe bleeding can be properly treated.

BRUISING

All children will go through a phase of having permanently bruised knees or shins! Parents often discover these at bath time when it is really too late to do anything about it. However, if you are presented with a bump soon after it has happened gentle pressure and/or an ice pack can reduce the swelling and subsequent bruising. Smoothing on a little arnica cream (available from most pharmacies) can also help. If bruising occurs frequently without known injury make an appointment to see your doctor.

Knocks on the head or face cause local swelling which develops at an alarming rate into a bump which can be the size of a plum. This is frightening if you haven't seen it happen before. Check for head injury symptoms (see page 222) and apply an ice pack (either ice cubes in a polythene bag placed in a tea towel or a packet of frozen peas in a tea towel!). The bump will slowly subside and leave a large bruise which will disappear over ten days or so.

BURNS

Action plan...

• Always treat a burn or scald with cold water.
• If possible immerse the burned area in cold water for at least ten minutes.
• Never apply any creams or greases.
• If hot liquid has spilt on to clothing remove the clothing immediately if possible. If not, wet it with cool or cold water then try to remove it. You must act quickly to avoid severe burns.
• If hands are affected do the same but then put the child's hand in a clean polythene bag while you contact the doctor.
• Apply clean wet wraps such as towels or even clingwrap to the burn while you transport the child to the surgery or casualty.
• You should contact your doctor, practice nurse or casualty department immediately for all but the most minor scalds.

DROWNING

When water enters the lungs it blocks the air passages and prevents the passage of oxygen from the air into the blood. If you come across someone who has just fallen into water they may be choking and there may be little to do except give a few firm slaps between the shoulder blades as described in the section on choking.

If the child seems to be unconscious, breathing may well have stopped.

Action plan...

• Hold the child with his head downwards

CHOKING

If a child accidentally inhales something from the mouth choking will result. Coughing nearly always dislodges whatever is causing the obstruction to the air passages but if this does not happen quickly then you will have to help to dislodge it.

ACTION PLAN...

● Look inside the mouth to see if it is possible to remove the object but do not put your fingers in to the back of the throat in case you push the object further down the windpipe. Then...

BABIES UNDER ONE YEAR:

● Lie the baby along your forearm or thigh with the head facing down.
● Give up to five firm slaps between the shoulder blades.
● If this does not work lie the baby on the floor on his back. Apply two fingers to an area a finger's width below the nipples in the middle of the chest and press down about 2cm.
● Keep repeating back slaps then chest thrusts.

● If the baby becomes unconscious do the chest thrusts five times then blow once gently into the lungs as instructed in the section on resuscitation.
● If you are on your own take your baby to the phone while you dial 999 but keep repeating these instructions until help arrives.

CHILDREN OVER ONE YEAR:

● Initially try to get the child to cough. Apply back slaps between the shoulder blades with the child leaning over your arm or the arm of a chair.
● If this does not work apply chest thrusts. Place the heel of the hand two fingers' width above where the ribs meet the breastbone. Press down five times.
● If this does not work try the back slapping again followed by chest thrusts.
● If the child becomes unconscious follow the instructions from the section on resuscitation. Make sure an ambulance is called and repeat these instructions until it arrives.

➤ RESUSCITATION

initially as breathing may start again when water drains out of the lungs.
● If there is still no sign of life it is important to start mouth to mouth respiration and heart massage right away.
➤ RESUSCITATION

ELECTRIC SHOCKS

Mild electric shocks cause pain and the child will jump away from the source of the shock and be quite distressed. Many electric shocks are much more serious than this and at best will cause burns and at worst cause the heart to stop beating.

Action plan...
● Firstly shut off the electricity supply at the socket or the mains before you touch the child.
● If the child is unconscious and not breathing call an ambulance and start heart massage and mouth to mouth respiration.
● If the child is still conscious check for burns. Electrical burns can be very deep and may be worse than they look. Treat as for burns and attend a casualty department for all but the most trivial burns.
➤ RESUSCITATION
➤ BURNS

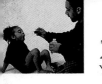

EYE INJURIES

If something has gone into a child's eye, whether it is sand, dust, soap or chemicals wash the eye with water. This will be difficult to do if you are on your own but you must do it right away even though the child will not like it. Dust can be washed away with water and chemicals will be diluted thereby reducing the risk of damage to the eye.

Action plan...
• Using a jug pour water on to the inside of the eye and use your other hand to keep the eyelids open.
• If you can see a piece of grit or other foreign body try to remove it with a cotton bud or a folded tissue.
• If you are worried at all attend a casualty department or your doctor's surgery. Do the same if there has been a direct blow to the eyeball. Noting the name of any chemical involved may be helpful.

FITS

➤ CONVULSIONS

FRACTURES

Fracture means a broken bone. It is usually caused by trauma from an injury although in the brittle bone disease (*Osteogenesis imperfecta*) bones may be broken with minimal trauma. If you suspect that your child may have a fracture then you should attend a casualty department. Suspicious signs are inability to bear weight in the case of the leg, ankle or foot, marked swelling or tenderness over one site and deformity is always highly suspicious. A child who does not seem to be using one arm or hand after an injury may have a fracture. In these cases

there is little point in attending your surgery and you should go straight to casualty where the doctors will assess the need for an x-ray.

A skull fracture is suspected if there is any abnormality, especially loss of consciousness, after a head injury, or if there is persistent vomiting.

HEAD INJURY

The rough and tumble of normal play can often lead to injury and head injury is common.

Contact the doctor if...
• the child has been unconscious or 'knocked out'
• the child has vomited after the injury
• you can see fluid coming from the ear or nose or there is bleeding from the ear
• there is unusual drowsiness
• the child is confused or cannot remember what has happened
• there is abnormal behaviour

Bumps on the head can cause swelling to arise at an alarming rate. Apply a cold compress and as long as the child is not showing any of the other signs listed above it is safe to wait and see. The lump will slowly reduce in size and the child should be back to normal in an hour or so.

NOSE BLEEDS

Nose bleeds can occur at any age, but are more likely if the nose is congested by a cold.

Pressure is the key word in any bleeding. In this case press just under the hard part of the bridge of the nose. Keep pressing for at least ten minutes and the bleeding will stop. Avoid tipping the head back. If bleeding repeatedly starts again after releasing the pressure, contact your doctor for advice. Once the bleeding is stopped the child should be kept calm – no running around for the next hour or so.

POISONING

Always contact your surgery or casualty department, whichever is likely to be the quicker, if your child has swallowed pills, medicine or household chemicals. Always check that the pills haven't spilled out of the bottle on to the floor but when you are as sure as you can be that the child has taken something, do not delay. If your child loses consciousness you may have to start resuscitation (see below). Your doctor may need to seek advice from the local Poisons Advice Centre so keep the bottle and tablets and try to give as much information as possible: the number of tablets taken, the name of the chemical from the label, the name of the manufacturer. You may think small quantities will probably do no harm, but check first.

RESUSCITATION

We can't say it enough. Remember the ABC of resuscitation: Airway, Breathing, Circulation.

AIRWAY

- When a child is found unconscious, the first thing to think about is the airway. Is it blocked?
- Look in the mouth and clear away any vomit or other obvious obstruction. Be careful not to push an object in further than it already is.
- Loosen tight clothing.

BREATHING

- Check for breathing – listen at the mouth, look for the chest moving, and see if you can feel breath on your cheek. Try not to spend more than ten seconds on this.
- If the child is not breathing, tilt the chin backwards slightly.
- Take a deep breath, put your mouth over the mouth, pinch the nose and breathe into the lungs. With smaller children you will have to put your mouth over their mouth and nose.
- Repeat this around 20 times per minute – once every three seconds.
- Check for circulation after the first two inflations

CIRCULATION

- It can often be difficult to find a baby's pulse. The best place is on the inside of the upper arm, midway between the shoulder and elbow. Place two fingers over the inside of the arm and press in towards the bone. If no pulse is present start heart massage.

HEART MASSAGE

- Place the child on a firm surface.
- Using your fingertips in small children, or the heel of your hand in older children, apply pressure to the bottom of the breastbone about 2cm below the nipples.
- Try to press about once per second with older children and slightly faster with babies and toddlers – around 100 times per minute. Press down between 1cm and 2cm.
- If you are alone give one breath to every five chest compressions. If you have help give two breaths for every five chest compressions applied by your helper.
- If you are alone, try to call 999 or shout for help after one minute. Then quickly return to resuscitation.
- If the child regains consciousness before the ambulance arrives place him in the recovery position.
- Do not leave the child alone.

To prevent such accidents always keep medicines locked away and don't put household chemicals in bottles which may attract children: lemonade bottles are a common culprit. As soon as they are old enough tell your children about not eating berries or toadstools. Always remember to clear up half-empty glasses after parties – remember that your children may well be up before you in the morning.

SPRAINS AND STRAINS

Sprains should be treated right away with pressure from a cold compress. Later the joint should be rested and supported with a crêpe or tubular bandage. If you are worried about the possibility of fracture you should attend a casualty department. Paracetamol can be given as can applied painkilling creams. Ask your pharmacist for advice.

A strain usually refers to a pulled muscle. This causes sudden pain over the muscle and there may be slight swelling. It is treated in the same way as a sprain.

SWALLOWED OBJECTS

Babies and toddlers love to put things in their mouths and can often end up swallowing them. With most coins and small toys the object will pass through the stomach and intestine and appear a few days later.

Follow the instructions given on page 221 about choking if the object seems to be causing breathing difficulty and follow the instructions on poisoning if the article is a pill or chemical. If the object is sharp or quite large call your doctor for advice.

➤ POISONING

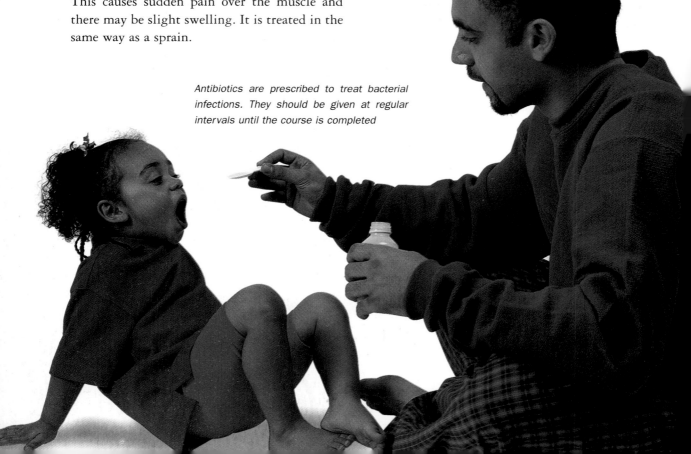

Antibiotics are prescribed to treat bacterial infections. They should be given at regular intervals until the course is completed

CHILDHOOD HEALTH: AN A–Z

Consult this list if you have any concerns about your baby's health and wellbeing. If you need any more help, ring your family doctor or health visitor.

ABDOMINAL PAIN

The 'abdomen' is any part of the body between the lower edge of the ribcage and the groin. Abdominal pain can occur with a wide range of illnesses from gastro-enteritis to diabetes and appendicitis. Pain can be constant or colicky – coming in waves. Colic pain often goes away completely between waves. The pain associated with 'tummy bugs' is often colicky and is due to spasms of the muscles of the intestines. Pains can also be associated with certain foods and the particular food may become obvious after two or three episodes.

In children there may be pain linked to diseases in other parts of the body such as tonsillitis or an ear infection. Children who suffer from sickle cell disease can get bouts of severe abdominal pain.

Appendicitis pain confuses many people. They know that it may move but don't know where. Essentially any organ in the abdomen which becomes inflamed may cause pain in the middle of the tummy. As the inflammation worsens the membrane which covers the organs, the peritoneum, becomes affected and the pain moves to the area of that organ – in the case of the appendix the right lower corner of the tummy. This is what is known as peritonitis. Most surgeons agree that appendices don't 'grumble' and recurrent abdominal pain is due to another cause such as constipation.

Abdominal pain is often a sign of an emotional upset such as bullying at school. This should always be suspected if a child often has tummy pain in the morning.

Children, especially younger children, may not have the vocabulary to explain if they don't feel well and tummy pain is simply their way of communicating that things are not right.

What you can do...
• If your child is old enough to tell you that her tummy hurts then she will probably be able to say where it hurts. Has anyone in the family or at nursery had diarrhoea? Does she complain when she passes urine? Is the urine smelly, cloudy or blood stained? Does her breath smell differently? Is she constipated? The doctor may ask questions like these.
• Try paracetamol at the recommended dose for the child's age. Paracetamol will not mask the symptoms of more serious problems but will often help the pain associated with diarrhoea or tonsillitis for example.
• A hot water bottle (not too hot of course!) can be soothing if placed on the tummy.
• If pain seems severe and has not been helped by paracetamol call the doctor for advice. For recurrent, less severe pain arrange to go into the surgery. If there is the possibility of collecting some urine for the doctor to test do so.

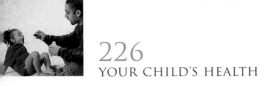

ADENOIDS

The adenoids are made of the same material as the tonsils and play a part in the body's defence against infection. They lie at the bottom of the Eustachian tubes which connect the inside of the ear with the back of the throat. However they cannot be seen from the mouth. Indications that they might be enlarged include snoring and frequent ear infections especially if this results in glue ear. In this case an ear, nose and throat specialist might advise removal of the adenoids. This is a simple operation.

➤ EAR INFECTION
➤ GLUE EAR

ALLERGIES

People, including children, can develop allergies to just about anything. Symptoms include a rash, itch, swelling, breathing difficulty, sneezing or watery eyes. People who are severely allergic to such things as bee stings may even collapse and become seriously ill. This is called anaphylaxis. This is rare in young children and is more likely if there has been a previous reaction to a substance.

Recently there have been worries about the apparent increase in the incidence of people allergic to nuts and nut products. Peanut (groundnut) oil is used as the main fat in many cakes, biscuits and other foods. Even worse than this is the fact that manufacturers of such products may use the same processing equipment to produce food which does not contain nuts but which may be contaminated by nuts. For this reason manufacturers warn consumers by stating on the packaging that the product may contain traces of nuts. This may make it difficult to buy processed food.

What you can do...

• Allergies may be caused by things we eat, things we put on our skin or things we breathe in. Minor reactions may need no treatment other than to stop using the substance involved.

• If there is facial swelling or breathing difficulty contact your doctor or casualty department at once.

• People who know they are allergic to bee stings or nuts can carry a special injection kit containing adrenaline to be given in case of anaphylaxis. This is also available for children.

• Less severe reactions can be treated with antihistamines. Your pharmacist will advise you but will usually recommend that children under the age of six see their GP first.

• New advice has been published on the subject of nut allergy. We are still not certain why so many people are becoming allergic to nuts but it may be that they are sensitised during pregnancy and breastfeeding. Therefore children, women who are pregnant and breastfeeding mothers who have a family history of allergy are advised to abstain from nuts, especially peanuts and groundnut oil. It is not recommended at the moment that all women avoid nuts.

ANAL FISSURE

A fissure is a small crack in the back passage which usually results from an episode of constipation. It is often extremely painful and may result in the child deliberately avoiding emptying the bowels because of the pain. Obviously this creates a vicious circle with further constipation.

Treatment involves using medicine to soften the bowel motion plus painkilling ointment to apply to the back passage if needed.

ANTIBIOTICS

Antibiotics are drugs which fight infection; doctors generally restrict the term to those that kill bacteria. Examples of bacterial infections include pneumonia and tonsillitis. The vast majority of winter ailments such as colds, flu, and chest infections are caused by a different type of organism called a virus and these do not respond at all to antibiotics.

When penicillin was first discovered it was effective against a wide range of bacteria, but as its use increased, bacteria were able to 'learn' to combat the antibiotic and it is now effective against only a limited number of bacteria. Research has produced dozens of new antibiotics since then but many have suffered the same fate. Doctors are becoming concerned at this escalating resistance to antibiotics and many now feel that we should avoid using them at all in infections that are known to be viral.

Since we have so few effective treatments for viral illnesses this means that diseases such as flu, colds, and most sore throats would be treated symptomatically (with drugs such as paracetamol for fever or antihistamines for stuffy noses and catarrh). By doing this we could keep effective antibiotic treatments for those infections which really need them. Doctors would still have to make a diagnosis in many cases. Most people can self-diagnose a cold, but any unexpected or worrying symptoms should be reported to a doctor. The doctor would then decide whether to issue over-the-counter remedies or to issue a prescription.

ASTHMA

A definition of asthma is a reversible narrowing of the air passages in the lungs. This causes wheeze (a whistling sound heard as the child breathes out) and, in younger children, a cough which is often more noticeable at night or after the child has been running around. The narrowing of the air passages is caused by inflammation in the lining of the passages, which in turn is caused by exposure to certain stimuli. These stimuli can differ from person to person. Common causes are dust from the coats of pets, cold air, infections and house dust mites which are present all over the house but especially in mattresses and pillows. One in five children in the UK now uses an inhaler at some time and the vast majority of children with asthma grow up to be healthy and able to take part in sports. Babies who have been breastfed for at least three months are less likely to suffer from wheeze than bottle-fed infants, as are babies who have not been given solid food until 15 weeks of age. These benefits last throughout early childhood.

Doctors seldom make the diagnosis of asthma from one episode of wheeze. Your doctor will look at the overall pattern of illnesses in each individual child so episodes of wheeze should be documented in the child's records and therefore the child should be taken to the surgery.

Asthma is treated by:
• Airway relaxer drugs given by inhaler (or syrup in young children) when wheeze is present.
• Prevention drugs, also given by inhaler, and taken regularly every day.

There are devices to help young children cope with inhalers and your doctor or practice nurse can show you how to use them. In severe attacks of wheeze doctors may prescribe oral steroid drugs even for very young children. Steroids are one of the most powerful treatments available for inflammation. Side effects are fairly rare if the steroid course is kept short.

What you can do...
• Avoid exposing children to cigarette smoke.
• Attend asthma clinics as often as your doctor recommends.
• Learn as much as you can so you understand the illness and its treatment.
• If a child becomes very breathless contact your doctor without delay.

ATHLETE'S FOOT

Athlete's foot is a fungal infection of the skin between the toes and sometimes spreading over the sole of the foot. It causes flaking and cracking of the skin and is often itchy.

What you can do...
• Fresh air is the easiest cure. Therefore avoid letting your child wear trainers all day.
• Buy socks which are made mainly of cotton so that they absorb sweat.
• Always dry toes thoroughly after baths.
• Use anti-fungal creams. Clotrimazole is available from the chemist or on prescription. There are also anti-fungal powders and sprays.

BED-WETTING

➤ SEE PAGE 215

BEHAVIOURAL PROBLEMS

This is difficult to define, as what may be one person's problem may be another's creative expression. However, most parents will see, from time to time, forms of behaviour in their children which they find difficult to cope with. Children learn appropriate behaviour gradually. For example, most two-year-olds do not take easily to sharing toys and this has resulted in many a toddler group bust-up. However the same children at the age of four may have realised that sharing can actually be fun. So it doesn't make sense to upset toddlers by trying to force them to share and it is better to try to distract one of them to play with something else. This is not pandering – it is simply exploitation of the natural course of events.

It is up to each family to set their own ground rules and to be consistent. Children will happily play one adult off against another if they think it might result in them getting their own way! And never ever make threats which you can't carry out. Children have amazingly good memories and won't be fooled twice.

If you feel that your child's behaviour is a problem take some time to think it through. Is it a problem just in your eyes or do other people agree? Is the behaviour causing danger to the child or others? Could it just be a phase that will pass and is therefore best ignored? Are you perhaps expecting too much for the age of your child? Are you giving mixed messages to your child? It is important to remember to praise the behaviour that you want so that your child receives positive messages from you.

Never forget that children can be affected by stress as much as adults and this can manifest itself as bad behaviour. So if there are changes in the household such as a new house, a new brother or sister, changes in routine such as going to nursery or even arguments in the family, then you should try to not get too upset when your child seems naughtier than usual.

BIRTHMARKS

So called 'stork marks' – a triangular red mark on the forehead and another red mark at the back of the neck – are very common, but fade over a few months and do not need treatment.

Strawberry naevi may grow over the first year or two but will have shrunk markedly by the time your child is seven years old. Parents are

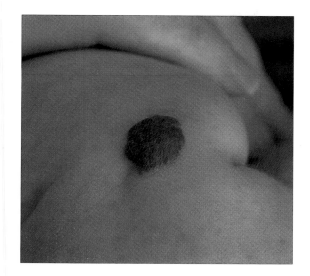

often alarmed by these as they can be a considerable size and can be raised up from the skin. However, unless they are causing secondary problems such as pressure on other tissues, it is better simply to wait for them to resolve on their own.

Port wine stains do not fade, but depending on the site and the size may be amenable to plastic surgery. They are flat and often a deep red colour.

In babies with dark skin there may be a pigmented area at the bottom of the back. These bruise-like marks are called Mongolian blue spots. Again they will fade in time but may take up to two years.

Babies may also have brown birthmarks like moles varying in size from a millimetre or two to a centimetre or more. They may also be hairy. These do not disappear.

BREAST ENLARGEMENT

A degree of breast enlargement is normal in newborn babies due to stimulation by the mother's female hormones before birth. It happens in both girls and boys and does not need treatment.

BREATH HOLDING

When some children become acutely upset or angry they may hold their breath for what seems like an unnaturally long time. You may find it happens more often if the child has been unwell or simply if they have had an active day and are very tired. It can be part of a tantrum and be a sign of sheer frustration. The child's body may become very stiff and tense and her face will be red or even purple. Most children will eventually cry but if they don't the attack may end with a loss of consciousness which will last for a few seconds or at the most up to a minute. This is extremely frightening for parents or carers but attacks end by themselves and no harm comes to the child.

What you can do...
• The first time it happens you will probably be too shocked to act quickly but always try to remain calm.
• Once you have seen an attack you may be able to predict the next one by the pattern of the child's behaviour. Give her a gentle shake, holding her arms to get her attention, or blow on to her face to try to stop the attack in its tracks. Then give her a firm cuddle.
• After the second or third attack you will probably be quite adept at predicting attacks. However, make an appointment at the surgery to confirm the diagnosis.

BREATHLESSNESS

Breathlessness can be caused by such things as infections, asthma or inhalation of a foreign body such as a peanut. If it has started suddenly or the child's lips are blue contact the doctor right away.

If breathing is rapid and/or shallow and the breathlessness is occurring at rest the advice is

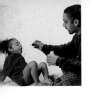

the same. If for any reason a doctor cannot be contacted take the child to a casualty department, preferably in a hospital with a children's department.

Children may become a bit more breathless than usual with a cough or cold. Noisy breathing can occur with, and may simply be due to, mucus in the nose or at the back of the throat. Babies and small children cannot clear their throats or blow their noses as we do but the mucus is not usually a problem. However, noisy breathing along with breathlessness will often need a doctor's advice. With a cold the breathing rate is no faster than normal unless the child has been exercising. Young children do not fake breathlessness so always take it seriously.

➤ ASTHMA
➤ BRONCHIOLITIS

BRONCHIOLITIS

Bronchiolitis is a viral infection which affects babies and children. It causes fast, shallow breathing, often with a high temperature. It can cause wheeze. It is not normally treatable by antibiotics although a doctor may prescribe them if a secondary infection is suspected. If there is breathing difficulty the child may have to go in to hospital.

If your baby or young child has rapid, shallow breathing seek advice from a doctor right away.

➤ BREATHLESSNESS
➤ VIRUSES

CEREBRAL PALSY

Cerebral palsy results from damage to the parts of the brain which control the body's movements and posture. This damage may occur before birth, during birth or during the first two years of life. The amount of damage caused may be slight or severe. The developing brain can be damaged by lack of oxygen, infections in the mother during pregnancy or a placenta which is not functioning properly. In many cases doctors are unable to find the exact cause. The blood vessels in the brain of premature babies are very fragile and are relatively easily damaged during labour and in the first few weeks of life, depending on the degree of prematurity. It follows that cerebral palsy is more common in very premature babies.

The damage may not always be evident at birth but may become obvious as the baby grows. Some of the tests done at the eight week screen check for cerebral palsy. However if parents are worried that their baby has not achieved any of the developmental milestones they should seek reassurance from their GP.

Children with cerebral palsy may need treatment throughout their childhood but parents should always be involved in the programme and in most cases will be able to help with exercises at home. Some sufferers of cerebral palsy may also have a mental handicap – another result of brain damage – but equally there may be no mental handicap whatsoever and the problem is purely a physical inability to control muscle movement.

CHEST INFECTIONS

A chest infection often follows a cold. Most are what doctors would call an acute bronchitis. Don't confuse this with the chronic (long-standing) bronchitis which affects smokers. In an otherwise healthy child acute bronchitis will last around a week, cause a cough with or without phlegm, and will gradually get better. The lungs have their own clearing mechanism and in a chest infection it is normal to have phlegm at the back of the throat in the morning. Coughing helps further to clear the phlegm. These infections do not usually need treatment with antibiotics.

Pneumonia is more serious. The child will often have a very high temperature, perhaps with severe shivering, and is generally very unwell. Pneumonia responds well to antibiotics.

What you can do...
• If your child has had a cold which has 'gone on to her chest' but she is otherwise well in herself, then it is worth waiting to see if she improves over 2–3 days. You can give a cough linctus at bedtime but avoid expectorants. Your pharmacist will advise you.
• If your child has a high temperature follow the instructions from the section on fever. If she still seems very unwell you should contact the doctor for advice.
➤ BRONCHIOLITIS
➤ COUGH

CHICKENPOX

➤ CHILDHOOD FEVERS (SEE PAGE 232)

CLEFT PALATE

Cleft palate and hare lip are linked conditions. When the palate forms in the fetus it forms in two parts which eventually fuse together. If any part of this fusion fails then a cleft palate or hare lip is the result. A hare lip is an obvious gap in the middle of the upper lip and a cleft palate is obvious only if you look inside the baby's mouth when you will see the gap in the roof of the mouth. Either can interfere with feeding. The action of sucking requires the baby to move the tongue along the palate and if there is a gap then this action is hampered. Plastic surgery is available for these children.

CLUB FOOT

This is also known as talipes and is caused by the feet being held in a fixed position in the womb so that the position is maintained after birth. It is more likely if the baby has been lying in the breech position. Talipes refers to a foot which curves inwards or outwards. The doctor who checks your baby after birth will check for talipes. In most cases the foot can be manipulated into the correct position and no treatment or very simple treatment is required. In the more severe cases surgery may be needed.

COLDS

The common cold is caused by viruses which are passed from person to person often by coughing and sneezing. The incubation period is short – just a few days. There is usually fever, a sore throat and muscle aches and pains which move from one part of the body to another. This can be followed by a cough with phlegm which lasts a few days, or an ear infection.

What you can do...
• See the section on fever and follow the same instructions. Antibiotics do not help colds or runny noses.

Contact the doctor if...
• the child is unduly listless. Fever causes listlessness so always try paracetamol first
• breathing is very fast or there is wheeze
• the child develops a cough without having had a cold or the cough goes on after the cold symptoms have gone
• there are signs from the checklist on meningitis
➤ CHILDHOOD FEVERS

COLD SORES

Cold sores are caused by a virus and appear as a sore spot around the mouth. They will often appear repeatedly in the same place. The virus can be passed to another person by contact so avoid kissing your child if you have an active cold sore. You can buy an anti-viral cream from the chemist which should be applied frequently as soon as you are aware that a cold sore is starting. This may help to diminish the frequency and severity of attacks.

COLIC

➤ ABDOMINAL PAIN
➤ SEE PAGE 37

CONGENITAL HIP DISLOCATION

If a joint is dislocated this means that one of the bones is out of place. In the case of the hip, which is a ball and socket joint, the 'ball' of the femur or thigh bone, is wholly or partially out of its 'socket' which is part of the pelvis.

Babies are checked at birth and at the eight week screen for dislocation of the hip. This condition, if missed, can cause problems with walking in later life. If a hip is found not to be dislocated but instead merely clicks when the hip is tested this will be followed up and investigations such as scans may be needed. Babies may have to wear a special splint for a while but most cope with these easily. Only very few will need an operation.

CONJUNCTIVITIS

Conjunctivitis can be caused by infection or allergy such as hay fever. Infective conjunctivitis is characterised by a discharge which causes a sticky eye. In allergies the eye tends to be watery. In both cases the eye is itchy, causing the child to scratch and the eye may be swollen. In the case of allergy the eye may swell so much that it appears closed.

What you can do...
• Bathe the eye with warm salty water.
• If the eye remains sticky make an appointment at the surgery.
• Infective conjunctivitis is very infectious so the child should have his own towel and nurseries often advise keeping the child at home until the infection is cleared.
• A very red eye, especially where the white of the eye is affected, should be seen that day by the doctor.
• Allergic conjunctivitis is treated by anti-histamines.

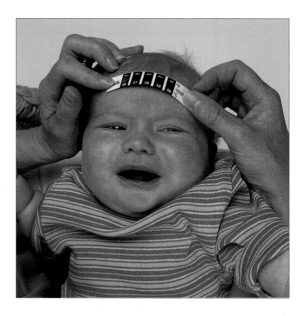

CHILDHOOD FEVERS

Nearly all of the childhood fevers are caused by viruses and so have no specific treatment. Always treat the fever with paracetamol and sponging (see page 216). Treat itchy rashes such

ILLNESS	INCUBATION PERIOD	EXCLUSION PERIOD	SYMPTOMS
Chickenpox	13–21 days	1–2 days before rash appears until spots have all crusted over Avoid contact with pregnant women in the first four months of pregnancy and near delivery	Crops of blisters mostly on the trunk
Erythema infectiosum Also known as 'fifth disease' and 'slapped cheek syndrome'	7–14 days	Nil	Mild illness 'Slapped cheek' appearance
Hand, foot and mouth disease	3–5 days	Feverish phase	Spots like tiny blisters on hands, feet and in the mouth (but often also on the backs of the legs, and on the buttocks)
Measles	8–13 days	A few days before the rash appears until 5 days after it goes	Fever, catarrh, initially like a very bad cold. Rash appears on the 3rd or 4th day and becomes widespread over the body. Children often very unwell
Mumps	14–21 days	7 days after the swollen glands appear	Fever, large swollen glands under the chin and in the cheek sometimes one side only
Roseola infantum	10 days	Nil	High temperature at first As the fever subsides over 1–3 days a fine spreading rash appears. This is short-lasting
Rubella (German measles)	14–21 days	7 days before the rash until 4 days after it appeared All pregnant women are offered a test for immunity to rubella. If in doubt, keep an infectious child away from a woman in early pregnancy	Usually a mild illness with a fine rash which may be more obvious after a bath
Scarlet fever	2–5 days	Until the child has had one day's treatment	Tonsillitis, a rash over the trunk and face and tongue described as a 'strawberry tongue'.The skin of the fingers may peel. This does need treatment with antibiotics
Whooping cough Also known as Pertussis	7–10 days	Up to 3 weeks after the fits of coughing start	Fever, catarrh, followed by coughing, with or without a 'whoop', which can go on for weeks. Needs antibiotics and the child is infectious up to 7 days after treatment

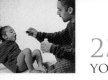

as chickenpox with calamine lotion or sponging with a solution of sodium bicarbonate (baking soda) in water and applied with cotton wool. The incubation period is the time from when the disease is first contracted by the child until the time when the first symptoms, usually fever, first appear. Even when the diagnosis is obvious, for example if you have nursed a child with chickenpox before and know the signs, the surgery should be notified. Public health departments keep a check on the incidence of many infectious illnesses in communities and your surgery should notify them of all cases.

CONSTIPATION

Most people will suffer from constipation at some time in their lives and children are no exception. Few people in developed countries eat enough roughage to keep their bowels emptying regularly throughout their lives. As well as roughage we need plenty of fluid to allow the fibre to swell and so stimulate the bowel to empty. The normal pattern varies from 2–3 times per day to once every two days. The pattern for breastfed babies can differ from those who are bottle-fed. Breastfed babies may dirty every nappy or may open their bowels very infrequently. They are less likely to develop constipation than babies fed on formula milk.

What you can do...
• Give your child more fibre. Oranges are excellent and you can also try other fruits, vegetables, peas and beans. Don't be tempted to add bran to a baby or toddlers diet as it may upset their system.
• Encourage your child to drink more but don't overdo the fizzy drinks or they may develop tummy pain.
• If this still doesn't work make an appointment at the surgery.

CONVULSIONS

The term convulsion means exactly the same as seizure or fit. A fit is caused by an abnormality of the electrical impulses in the brain. It may start with the person staring into space or with small repetitive movements. The person may fall on to the ground and the movements may become more jerky. He may be quite stiff and may salivate. There might be moaning noises and a change in colour of the skin to a dusky blue colour. When the jerking stops the child will be drowsy for a while and may seem confused.

All of this is very frightening to an onlooker who has not seen a fit before. However it is important to remain calm and not to panic.

In the event of a fit...
• Move him away from any potentially dangerous object.
• There is no need to hold the tongue or put anything into the mouth.
• When the jerking stops move him into the recovery position.
• If the child continues to fit for more than a minute call the doctor. Also call the doctor if the fit stops but starts again soon after.
• If the child has never had a fit before call the doctor.
➤ RESUSCITATION

Febrile convulsions
Fits may occur when a child's temperature is very high. Children over five are less likely to be affected and the risk reduces with age. Sometimes the fit may be the first indication that a child is ill. To prevent a fit it is crucial that efforts to keep the temperature down continue until the fever 'breaks'. This may not happen until 2–3 days after an illness has started. Follow page 216, Treating a Fever, and

try to get help for part of the day at least. You will find nursing a sick child exhausting.

Always call the doctor. He or she may advise that admission to hospital would be best, but if there is an obvious cause this may not be necessary and treatment may be given at home.

During the fit follow the instructions as for convulsions above. Make sure that you have given the correct amount of paracetamol and keep the child cool. Tepid sponge until the temperature comes down.

COUGH

Most children will develop a cough after a cold. This can be a dry cough or a cough which causes phlegm or sputum to be coughed up. The lungs are very good at clearing themselves and most healthy children will get over a cough in about a week. Most coughs are caused by viruses and antibiotics don't help.

Contact the doctor if...
• the child is also very breathless
• the child appears generally very unwell, with a very high temperature or severe shivering
• the cough started after the child choked on food

Otherwise make an appointment if...
• the cough lasts more than a week and does not seem to be improving
• the cough is worse at night or comes on after exercise. This can be a sign of asthma

Your pharmacist can advise on cough remedies for night time to allow the child to get some sleep. Avoid expectorants at night.

Parents – stop smoking! Passive smoking can cause chronic cough in childhood.

Coughs can often alarm parents. Children may appear to have difficulty coughing up phlegm and will often cough throughout the night. You can help your child by patting him on the back or letting him inhale steam. (Do take care with hot water around babies!) In most cases of cough where the child is not otherwise unwell the cause is a virus, the chest is clear when the doctor examines it, and there is little else to be done until the chest clears itself of phlegm (by coughing!).

CRADLE CAP

Cradle cap is a condition which affects the scalp of babies and which causes flaking and a build up of yellowish crusts on the scalp. It does not upset the baby but parents are understandably concerned because it is unsightly.

What you can do...
• In mild cases use baby shampoo.
• If this doesn't work try applying olive oil at night and washing it off in the morning. This will help in almost all cases but it needs to be continued for some time to keep the scalp clear.
• Ask your health visitor for advice.

CROUP

Croup is a viral illness which results in a child having difficulty breathing in. Doctors can often make the diagnosis over the phone as there is a very characteristic noise a little like a sea lion barking.

What you can do...
• Give paracetamol for any associated fever.
• Try steam. You can do this by switching on a shower or by putting saucepans of boiling water on the hob or if you have a tumbler dryer dampen some towels and put them in.
• If there is no improvement after 20 minutes call the doctor.

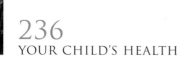
DEAFNESS

Babies have a hearing test at eight months of age. If deafness is suspected the test will often be repeated and if the health visitor is still suspicious she will arrange further testing. Parents are very good judges of their children's hearing and audiograms are easy to arrange if there is any suspicion of deafness. Repeated ear infections and glue ear may lead to hearing loss and subsequent delay in language development so make an appointment at your surgery if you are worried. Hearing may be temporarily reduced by a cold.

DIABETES

Diabetes mellitus is a disease affecting the pancreas gland in the abdomen. This gland produces the substance insulin which helps the body use up the sugar which comes from our diet. If there is insufficient insulin glucose builds up in the bloodstream and this can cause problems for many of the organs of the body.

Diabetics have to inject themselves with insulin on a regular basis. Insulin cannot be given by mouth. Parents are often concerned at the thought of either giving their child injections or the thought of the child giving injections to himself. It is always surprising how even young children cope. If your child is diagnosed with diabetes mellitus it is vitally important that he attends all check-ups and that together you learn to keep the strictest possible control over his blood glucose to avoid complications in later life.

A 'hypo' refers to an episode of hypoglycaemia or low blood sugar. This may happen if a diabetic has had his normal dose of insulin but for some reason, often a stomach upset, has not had his normal food intake. The child may be sweaty and sleepy or even confused. It is vital that he is given sugar in any form although special tablets are available which are convenient to carry around. An untreated hypo may result in unconsciousness and then it is essential to call a doctor.

You may have come across diabetics who use oral tablets. These are usually only suitable for people who have developed diabetes in later life. Children with diabetes will nearly always need insulin to gain control over their blood sugar.

DIARRHOEA

Diarrhoea means frequent and/or loose bowel motions. It can be due to infections or to intestinal diseases such as colitis (rare in young children) or an inability to digest certain foods.

A small sample of stool can be sent to the laboratory to test for infection in any case of diarrhoea lasting longer than a few days. Prolonged diarrhoea should always be investigated and so you should make an appointment at your surgery.
➤ GASTRO-ENTERITIS

DIPHTHERIA

Diphtheria is rarely seen in the UK nowadays partly as a result of the immunisation programme which ensures that babies receive immunisation to diphtheria from the age of eight weeks. The illness does not begin acutely and there may not be much of a fever. However it worsens as it progresses and the characteristic feature is a grey membrane in the throat. The fact that it is rare in Britain should not stop parents immunising their children as it is still seen in other countries.

DRY SKIN

The skin of babies and children can become dry very easily and this may cause itching and flakiness. In mild cases use baby lotion. If it still seems to disturb the child then it is worth making an appointment at the surgery as the child may be suffering from eczema.

➤ ECZEMA

EARACHE

Earache is common after a cold and can be a sign of an ear infection.

What you can do...
• Always give paracetamol at the stated dose for the age of the child.
• Comfort the child. Children can become very distressed by the pain of earache.
• If the pain continues after giving paracetamol see your doctor at the next available surgery. Antibiotics are sometimes prescribed for earache but they do not relieve pain. If there are worrying symptoms other than the earache phone your doctor for advice.

EAR INFECTION

Ear infections often occur after a cold. Most are caused by viruses. The area infected is called the middle ear and connects with the rear nasal passages by way of tubes called the Eustachian tubes. At the bottom of these tubes lie the adenoids. Therefore, if a child seems to contract a lot of ear infections and the hearing becomes affected she may be referred to an ear, nose and throat surgeon who might consider removing the adenoids. Hearing will often be temporarily reduced during an ear infection.

Follow directions as for earache. Ear infections sometimes need to be treated by antibiotics. However they are not regarded as a medical emergency and an appointment should be made at the surgery.

Many parents worry about a perforated eardrum. This can happen with an ear infection and may result in a yellow or green discharge from the ear. Perforated eardrums in children heal up very well and do not usually cause long-term problems with hearing. They may even help earache because of the release of pressure. Antibiotics do not prevent perforated eardrum.

Young children often develop ear infections, tonsillitis and chest infections. When deciding on whether or not to remove adenoids (and tonsils) ear, nose and throat surgeons will take into consideration deafness and days lost from school. Adenoid removal does not prevent colds or throat infections.

➤ ADENOIDS

EAR WAX

It is normal to have some wax in the ears. Never push a cotton bud into the ear canal as you can actually increase the amount of wax produced. Clean only the outside of the ear.

EATING PROBLEMS

Most children will go through phases where they seem to eat very little. It can often be quite amazing how little they can eat and still maintain their body weight!

What you can do...
• Don't worry. If you need reassurance ask your health visitor to weigh your child. If the child's body weight is within the accepted band for their age and height there is no need to worry. We all want our children to eat a balanced diet but the worst thing you can do is engage in warfare at the tea table. All children enjoy finding ways to exert some authority as they go through toddlerhood and if they find that mummy gets in a tizz when they don't eat their greens then suddenly it is fun to not eat greens.

It can be exasperating to spend time preparing a meal only to find that he hasn't taken a mouthful but you must keep calm!

• Eating should be an enjoyable social occasion for the whole family. If possible sit down at the table together in the evenings. Give the reluctant eater small portions and allow plenty of time for him to try the food.

• Don't cajole but if he remains reluctant clear the table. However don't throw the food out unless it is going to be inedible later. Then don't give in to requests for sweets or snacks.

• It all sounds so simple but it is incredibly difficult to put into practice. Everyone who cares for your child has to be consistent or your plan will be doomed to failure.

ECZEMA

Eczema and dermatitis mean the same thing – inflamed skin. The tendency for the skin to become dry and inflamed may be inherited and other family members may also have asthma or hay fever. Eczema is a very itchy condition and children will often scratch until their skin appears very red and raw. This type of eczema often starts in the first or second year of life. It is less common in breastfed babies. Another type of eczema can also arise from contact with an irritant such as bleach or washing powder.

What you can do...
• Avoid obvious irritants.

• Use plenty of moisturiser – not the perfumed variety. These are available on prescription for eczema sufferers. Moisturising the skin is the crucial element of eczema treatment. In severe cases it may have to be done several times a day.

• Make an appointment at the surgery if moisturisers fail to stop the skin drying out and it becomes red and sore.

ENURESIS

➤ BED-WETTING

EYE INFECTION

➤ CONJUNCTIVITIS

FIFTH DISEASE

➤ CHILDHOOD FEVERS

FITS

➤ CONVULSIONS

FLAT FEET

Children naturally tend to have flat feet compared to adults who have an arch in their instep. It is often the case in children that no arch can be seen at all. However when the child stands on tiptoe you will often see the arch then. Flat feet are one of the orthopaedic conditions which used to be treated with such things as insoles and even special shoes. Over the years it became apparent that many of these treatments had little effect on the eventual outcome and therefore they were abandoned. Flat feet only very rarely need to be treated.

FORESKIN

The foreskin is normally tight at birth and should not be pulled back. Usually by the time the child is three the foreskin can be gently pulled back, but if you feel that it is too tight after this then make an appointment at the surgery. The doctor may diagnose phimosis and circumcision may be recommended.

Balanitis is an infection under the foreskin which causes inflammation sometimes with a discharge of pus. It may be treated by antibiotics.

GASTRO-ENTERITIS

This is an infection of the digestive system which often starts with vomiting and leads to diarrhoea. The exact course of the illness varies depending on the particular 'bug' causing it. Most communities will have minor 'epidemics' of vomiting and diarrhoea from time to time. You may hear of other children being off nursery or school with a 'tummy bug'.

What you can do...
• Give plenty of fluids. The real danger with these infections is dehydration and young babies are most at risk. Even if a child is vomiting you must persevere with fluids.
• During the vomiting phase you can withhold food if the child does not seem hungry.
• During the diarrhoea phase food can be given but again fluids are your top priority.
• Give paracetamol for fever if required.
• Don't give diarrhoea mixtures to very young children as many contain chemicals similar to morphine. These can have drastic side effects for babies and small children. At this age diarrhoea can often drag on for days on end and if it is very prolonged doctors may occasionally prescribe a safe preparation. However, in the early stages it is best simply to persevere with fluids. Doctors rarely prescribe medicine to stop vomiting.
• Sachets of rehydration powders are sometimes given to babies and children with vomiting or diarrhoea. These contain salts which can be lost during these illnesses. These powders will not stop vomiting or diarrhoea. They are prescribed only to stop dehydration. In most tummy bugs drinks such as dilute squashes will do just as well.
• Wash your hands. These illnesses are passed

on more readily if there is poor hygiene so always wash your hands after going to the toilet and before handling food.

Contact the doctor if...
• vomiting is persistent and you are worried about dehydration. Look for: a dry mouth or tongue, a sunken fontanelle, dry nappies
• the child is very listless or floppy
• you see projectile (very forceful) vomiting

GERMAN MEASLES (RUBELLA)

➤ CHILDHOOD FEVERS

GLUE EAR

After an ear infection the middle ear will usually clear itself of fluid and will return to being full of air. However in a few cases fluid will remain and this can prevent the ear from transmitting sound waves – deafness can result. We call this situation glue ear. As there is no longer any infection, antibiotics will not work. If the ear does not clear itself the child may be referred to an ear, nose and throat surgeon who may insert grommets in to the ear drum. Grommets are tiny tubes which sit in the ear drum and allow air back in to the middle ear. The grommets may dislodge some months later and you might find that one has fallen out. Hopefully by this time the glue ear will be cured. Sometimes the adenoids will be removed at the same time as the grommets are put in.
➤ ADENOIDS

HAND, FOOT AND MOUTH DISEASE

➤ CHILDHOOD FEVERS

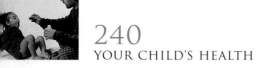

HARE LIP

➤ CLEFT PALATE

HAY FEVER

Hay fever is an allergy to pollen which causes watery, itchy eyes, a watery discharge from the nose, and sneezing. The season of allergy extends from March until September depending on which particular pollens the sufferer is allergic to. Treatment in children is usually by antihistamine syrups or nasal sprays. Some children respond to homoeopathic treatment.

HEADLICE

Most children will pick up headlice at some point in their lives. Contrary to popular belief they are not a sign of poor hygiene.

Don't wait for the telltale sign of scratching: be your own nit-nurse and check weekly for any sign of headlice. The eggs or nits are often seen in the hair behind the ears, under the fringe, or at the nape of the neck. Dead eggs look a bit like dandruff but are stuck firmly to the hair; unhatched eggs are darker. Comb regularly with a fine tooth comb which will help to get rid of nits and also damage adult lice. 'Leave in' conditioner on wet hair makes this easier.

Most headlice lotions sold by pharmacists contain malathion. Many of these products have an alcohol base and can adversely affect asthmatics. Because of recent worries about the safety of malathion many people have turned to dilute preparations of tea tree oil sold in herbalists shops. Many of the headlice shampoos are ineffective because headlice have become resistant to them. A better option may be to use preparations of essential oils as a repellent – ask your pharmacist.

Adults can carry headlice without realising.

They cannot hop, jump, or fly from one head to another; they have to be passed by contact.

HEART MURMURS

When a doctor listens to the heart she can hear two sounds, one after the other in succession. These are the normal heart sounds. If there is an extra sound then this is usually called a murmur. A murmur is the sound of the blood flowing through the heart. Heart murmurs may be normal at certain stages of development and there is often a murmur when there is a fever due to the blood rushing through the heart. However if your doctor is unsure why the murmur is present she may refer your child for a second opinion from a specialist.

HEAT-STROKE

Never allow your children to become over-exposed to the sun. At best they will suffer mild sunburn. At worst they will develop heat-stroke and may be more at risk of skin problems in later life. Use sun hats and T-shirts to keep the sun from their skin and if they want to swim use a high factor sun block and apply it regularly.

The symptoms of heat-stroke are headache, nausea and vomiting, and drowsiness. The child may seem confused and may be dehydrated.

What you can do...
• Give paracetamol for the headache.
• Give plenty of drinks.
• Let the child lie down for a while.
• If you are worried about excessive drowsiness or confusion call your doctor for advice.

HERNIAS

A hernia means a part of the digestive system is lying outside the cavity of the abdomen where it should be. The commonest hernia is a protrusion of the intestine through the wall of the abdomen at a point where the muscles have a weakness. This may be in the groin or around the navel. Some herniae may need surgical treatment to prevent them from becoming 'strangulated' – stuck outside the abdomen.

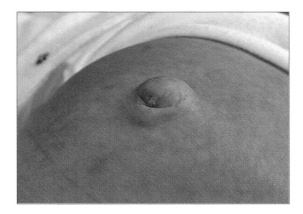

IMMUNISATIONS

The current recommendations for immunisation of children are as follows:

At two, three and four months
• DTP (Diphtheria, tetanus, pertussis)
• Polio
• Hib (*Haemophilus influenzae* meningitis)
Hib and DTP are given in one injection and polio as drops in the baby's mouth.

At 12–15 months
• Measles, mumps and rubella (MMR)

3–5 years
• Booster diphtheria, tetanus and polio
• MMR second dose

10–14 years (or earlier if there is exposure to TB)
• BCG

13–18 years
• Booster diphtheria, tetanus and polio
Immunisations may be postponed if the baby is suffering from an acute illness when the immunisation is due. However, snuffles or a cough where the baby does not have a temperature and is otherwise well will not usually delay an immunisation. Your practice nurse will advise you.

Booster doses may not be given if there has been a severe reaction to a previous dose. It is normal for babies to be grumpy and even have a mild fever after an immunisation. It is also normal for there to be some swelling at the injection site. Always make sure you have paracetamol in the house when your baby has been immunised. Give it at the recommended dose for the age of the child and you will find that it will help your baby to settle.

Children who suffer from diseases which affect their immune system will not usually be given live vaccines such as polio.

Immunisations will not usually be postponed in premature babies. This means they will start at eight weeks after birth just the same as babies born at term.

Recent reports linking MMR vaccine to autism and inflammatory diseases of the bowel such as Crohn's disease have not been proven.

The Hib vaccine is given to prevent meningitis caused by the organism *Haemophilus influenzae*, which before the introduction of the vaccine caused a number of cases of meningitis each year. However, this vaccine does not prevent meningitis by the organism meningococcus which unfortunately still causes a number of deaths in children each year. Meningococcal vaccine is given to contacts of cases of meningococcal meningitis.

For advice on travel vaccines make an appointment with your practice nurse well before the date of travel. Travel agents vary

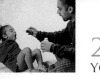

enormously with regard to the reliability of the information they give. If you have booked a holiday to a risky area immunise your family according to the current recommendations. Don't take chances simply to avoid jabs. Diseases such as typhoid or hepatitis A can be serious in adults, never mind small children.

IMPETIGO

Impetigo is an infection of the skin, often the face, which is characterised by yellow crusty patches around inflamed areas on the skin. It is infectious. It often requires an antibiotic so if it doesn't clear up in a day or two make an appointment at the surgery.

INFLUENZA

Influenza is an illness caused by viruses. The obvious features of influenza (or flu as most people call it) are very high temperatures and muscle aches. The temperature can be so high that the person feels unable to get out of bed but this phase of the illness is usually quite short lasting – just a couple of days or so. This is followed by exhaustion which can go on for a few days and there may be complications such as a chest infection or blocked sinuses.

What you can do...
• There is no cure for flu. The temperature should be treated with paracetamol according to the age of the child. If there are any additional symptoms which cause concern contact the doctor for advice.

INTOEING

This often becomes obvious as the child learns to walk and the toes are seen to point inwards sometimes causing the child to stumble and fall over. However, it rights itself as the child grows and no treatment is needed.

JAUNDICE

Jaundice means that the skin has a yellow tinge to it and the whites of the eyes are also yellow. This is due to an excess of a pigment called bilirubin, which is sometimes measured if a newborn is particularly jaundiced. A degree of jaundice is to be expected in the first few days but may be more severe if a baby is premature. Treatment is by light therapy (phototherapy).

Jaundice at any other time in a baby or child must be dealt with by a doctor.

JOINT PAINS

Joint pains may be acute (short-lived) as in flu and other viral illnesses, or may be chronic (long-standing) as in arthritis. Arthritis is rare in children. More common is a range of conditions which affect the growing points of bones. These can be quite painful but are rarely serious and disappear when the bones stop growing. Nevertheless if a child complains persistently of joint pains you should take him to your doctor. Contact the doctor right away if a child is suddenly unable to put weight on one leg or does not seem to be using one arm.

KIDNEY INFECTIONS

Kidney and bladder infections (cystitis) are caused by bacteria getting into the tube which empties the bladder (the urethra) and travelling upwards into the bladder and kidneys. These bacteria are usually ones which live in the skin around the groin area and most come from the bowel. However, urine infections are not a sign of poor hygiene and are not infectious.

What you can do...
• There may be a fever. The child may complain of stinging when passing urine. Cloudy or bloodstained urine indicate infection.
• If these are present contact the doctor who may prescribe an antibiotic.
• Give the child plenty of fluids.

KNOCK-KNEES

Knock-knees mean that when the child stands with his knees together there is a gap between the feet. Whether or not treatment is required depends entirely on the size of the gap and parents are often surprised that treatment is not given. However this is a condition which will often right itself and opinion is consistent between orthopaedic surgeons about the degree of deformity which requires treatment.

The same can be said of the opposite condition bow legs, where the child stands with his ankles together but has a gap between the knees. This used to be seen often as a result of the condition rickets which resulted from a deficiency of calcium or vitamin D. Nowadays this condition is rare and few cases of bow legs require treatment.

LARYNGITIS

Laryngitis is an inflammation of the larynx or voice box and causes either hoarseness or croup in young children. It often follows a cold and is usually caused by viruses so antibiotics are rarely of any help. In an adult or older child doctors will usually advise resting the voice but try telling that to a toddler!

If there's no evidence of croup, with its characteristic cough, laryngitis will usually get better gradually by itself and in a child who is otherwise well there is no need to do anything about hoarseness which lasts a few days. If it

goes on for longer than this make an appointment at the surgery.

LIMP

A limp occurs when there is pain in the foot, leg, hip or back and will usually arise as a result of an injury. If a fracture is suspected then the child must go to a casualty department. Lesser injuries may cause sprains and strains (see page 224). However young children do not fake limps, at least not for very long. Therefore any limp which arises without injury should be investigated and the child should be taken to the next available surgery.

MEASLES

➤ CHILDHOOD FEVERS

MENINGITIS

This is the one which worries all parents and doctors alike. Cases are still missed because the symptoms can vary from case to case. The organisms are passed from person to person by droplet spread (like a cold). The incubation period is 2–3 days. There is usually a fever, the child is often off colour and there may be vomiting. There may be a rash early on which doctors would call non-specific – it doesn't have obvious signs of any particular rash and the spots go pale (blanch) on pressure. Later on the rash of meningitis is quite unmistakable. The spots may be pink or purple but the obvious feature is that they do not blanch. You can try this yourself. If you take a tumbler and press it down on many skin blemishes you will see them go pale. If you try it on a mole there is no change in its colour. Meningitis spots are like this. If you ever see this kind of rash on an adult or a child you must get medical help immediately. If there is any delay in contacting a GP you should take your child to a casualty department preferably in a hospital with a children's ward.

Other signs are a stiff neck or back, unusual drowsiness or a change in the sound of a baby's cry. Older children may complain of pain when they look at a light (photophobia). The child may be very irritable.

One of the problems with meningitis is that the early signs are the same as those of a fever. On an average night on call a GP may see several children with fevers. Although your doctor will think about meningitis and probably test for it, a child who is in the early stages may not show the signs until some hours later. Don't be afraid to ask your doctor about the signs to look for and if your child's condition seems to be deteriorating call back. Thankfully meningitis is extremely rare and if we all remain vigilant we can make it rarer still.

Look for these signs of meningitis:
- severe headache
- high temperature
- stiff neck
- vomiting
- drowsiness
- sensitivity to light
- rash as described above

MOLLUSCUM CONTAGIOSUM

This appears as a crop of small, shiny, raised spots often appearing as a small group on one part of the body. It is mildly infectious and is passed through close contact. It is treated for cosmetic reasons if the spots are on a conspicuous area but treatment is not necessary if the crop is small and the spots are not bothering the child as the spots will go by themselves eventually.

MUMPS

➤ CHILDHOOD FEVERS

NAPPY RASH

This is caused by the skin of the nappy area coming into contact with urine or faeces and may be complicated by thrush in some cases.

What you can do...
- Leave the nappy off whenever possible. Fresh air will help their bottom heal.
- Change nappies often. It doesn't matter whether you use terries or disposables, the same rule applies.
- Apply small amounts of barrier cream. Large quantities can affect the absorption of disposable nappies.
- Be extra cautious at any time when your baby's diet is changing or if your child develops diarrhoea or loose bowel movements.
- Use baby lotion, lotion wipes or gentle baby soap to clean the skin.
- If all this has failed, your doctor can prescribe an anti-fungal cream to apply to the skin.

➤ SEE PAGE 59

PERTUSSIS

➤ CHILDHOOD FEVERS

PNEUMONIA

Pneumonia is an inflammation of the lungs, usually caused by an infection. The child may have a cold and a fever, and will be breathless with rapid shallow breathing even when he is asleep. See your doctor. Some children need admitting to hospital, some simply need antibiotics.

PRICKLY HEAT

This occurs during hot weather and is made worse by exposure to the sun. It is extremely itchy and there may be redness of the skin.

You can treat it with antihistamines or hydrocortisone cream 1%, available from your pharmacist. Always remember the golden rules with these creams: use sparingly, don't apply to the face unless advised to do so by your doctor, and stop using it as soon as the condition gets better.

PYLORIC STENOSIS

The pylorus is the exit from the stomach into the first part of the intestines, the duodenum. Stenosis is the medical term for a tightening, so pyloric stenosis means that the outflow from the stomach is partially blocked. This may cause projectile vomiting – vomiting that is so forceful that it travels a distance and may even hit the opposite wall of the room! Babies with pyloric stenosis may need to have a small operation to relieve the blockage. This condition almost always becomes apparent in the first eight weeks of life.

RASHES

Skin rashes can be caused by infections or allergies or by diseases which affect the skin such as eczema.

An infection-related rash will usually be accompanied by a fever and signs that the child is ill such as catarrh or just being off colour. Allergies may produce a mild fever but this is rare. The child usually appears very well and this rash is often intensely itchy. It may take the form of red spots which seem to run into each other or urticaria which may look like a nettle rash or have raised blotches with paler centres.

Eczema is also itchy but the skin is often unusually dry and may be painful.
➤ CHILDHOOD FEVERS

ROSEOLA INFANTUM

➤ CHILDHOOD FEVERS

RUBELLA

➤ CHILDHOOD FEVERS

SCABIES

Scabies is caused by a tiny mite which burrows in to the skin. It is very infectious and causes intense itching. It tends to be worse in areas where the mite is trapped such as waistbands and also between the fingers. It is treated by a cream or lotion which is available on prescription or from your pharmacist.

SCARLET FEVER

➤ CHILDHOOD FEVERS

SHINGLES

Shingles is rare in children. It is caused by the chickenpox virus so you can't have shingles until you have had chickenpox. The virus affects one skin nerve so it appears on one side of the body only and causes a crop of blisters very similar to chickenpox but in a cluster. It can be very painful so see your doctor.

SICKLE CELL DISEASE

Sickle cell disease is an inherited condition found in people of West African or Afro-Caribbean descent. The substance which transports oxygen around the body is called haemoglobin. People with sickle cell disease have a different type of haemoglobin which takes on a different shape when it gives up its oxygen to the tissues. The red cells containing the haemoglobin become sickle shaped. This results in them being broken down more quickly than normal in the spleen and so sufferers may frequently become anaemic. Also the abnormally shaped cells can cause blockages of blood vessels which leads to episodes of pain in the limbs or abdomen. Episodes may last a few days and should be treated with painkillers such as paracetamol.

SLAPPED CHEEK SYNDROME

➤ CHILDHOOD FEVERS

SORE THROATS

Sore throats can be caused by inflammation of the tonsils (tonsillitis), the larynx (laryngitis) or the pharynx (pharyngitis). The tonsils are the spongy looking areas on either side of the arch as you look at the back of the throat, the pharynx is the bit beyond the arch – the back of the throat – and the larynx you can't see because it is too far down but you know you have laryngitis if you are hoarse. Younger children may develop croup if their larynx is affected.

All sore throats may be accompanied by a fever, nasal congestion and a cough. There will also be swollen glands – see separate section. Tonsillitis will generally be the worst of the three and causes a child to be generally unwell.

What you can do...
• First of all treat as for a fever. If the child is otherwise OK she may not need to see a doctor and you will be able to treat her yourself.
• The vast majority of sore throats are caused by viruses. Antibiotics make absolutely no

difference to the progress of the disease. Doctors may decide to treat tonsillitis with antibiotics but pharyngitis does not respond to antibiotics. Thankfully it only lasts a few days.
• In older children painkilling lozenges may help – ask your pharmacist.
• All sore throats cause pain on swallowing but if the child has difficulty in swallowing contact your doctor.

SQUINT

A child's eye may squint inwards (convergent squint) or outwards (divergent squint). As a squint would usually cause double vision the brain copes with this by suppressing the image from one eye. This can become permanent and so it is important to seek advice if you even suspect your child may have a squint.

Either your doctor, child health clinic or optician can refer your child to an orthoptist who is a specialist in squints.

SUNBURN

Treat sunburn with calamine lotion and cool baths. Paracetamol is also helpful for pain.
➤ HEAT-STROKE

SWOLLEN GLANDS

The glands which most people refer to when they describe swollen glands are those under the chin. These glands are known to doctors as lymph nodes and they are part of the body's defences against infection. There are lymph nodes all over the body, some just under the skin and some deep inside the body. As soon as an infection is contracted the local glands start to work. In some viral infections, glands will swell all over the body. Swollen glands on their own do not constitute a diagnosis and your doctor would try to identify the cause of the swollen glands. In most cases this will be a virus which requires no treatment other than that for fever. The glands will usually reduce in size after a week or two to the size of a baked bean. Glands which remain enlarged for longer than this should be checked by a doctor.

TALIPES

➤ CLUB FOOT

TEETHING

➤ SEE PAGE 116

THREADWORM

Threadworms, like headlice, are a common problem of childhood and are not a sign of poor hygiene. The worms are white and about half an inch long and live in the bowels. They come out of the back passage at night to lay their eggs on the skin when they cause the child to have an itchy bottom. The child scratches, eggs get stuck under the nails where they stay until the child passes them on to someone else the next day. Pretty disgusting really but easily treated!

What you can do...
• Anyone over the age of two can take a dose of piperazine 100mg, available from your chemist or on prescription. It is sensible to treat the whole family and repeat the dose after 10 days if worms are still seen in the bowel motions.
• Teach your child to wash her hands often.
• Keep your child's nails short.

THRUSH

➤ SEE PAGE 59

TONSILLITIS

➤ SORE THROATS

TOOTHACHE

Toothache is often caused by dental caries or tooth decay. To help prevent decay from occurring, children should be taught to brush their teeth from an early age but should be helped until you are certain that they are capable of doing it thoroughly by themselves.

Make sure you are registered with a dentist. They're only obliged to offer emergency treatment to patients already registered with them.

What you can do...
• Always try paracetamol at the recommended dose for the age of the child. This will be sufficient for most mild toothaches.
• Contact your dentist if toothache is severe. After surgery hours you will usually get an answering machine giving you instructions on how to contact the dentist. If you are requested to leave a message the dentist will ring you back later. All NHS dentists have to provide an emergency service to their patients.
• If you do not have a dentist telephone your local casualty department where there may be an emergency dental service the next day.
• Your GP does not have the means to make a diagnosis in dental problems and will only provide pain relief in an absolute emergency where a dentist cannot be contacted. Because they have no training in dental problems GPs will not usually prescribe antibiotics unless the diagnosis of abscess is very obvious.

TOXOCARIASIS

This infection is caused by an organism called Toxocara and is picked up from the faeces of dogs and cats where the organism's eggs are found. This disease may cause blindness but it is preventable. All pets should be wormed regularly. Ask your vet for advice. If you have a dog do make sure that you clean up behind it.

TOXOPLASMOSIS

Toxoplasmosis is an infection caused by an organism called a protozoan. This may be found in raw or undercooked meat and also in the faeces of cats and sometimes dogs. In the vast majority of cases infection does not produce any symptoms except for swollen glands and patients eventually recover.

However toxoplasmosis, if picked up by a pregnant woman, can be passed on to her baby and this can have devastating effects such as visual impairment, epilepsy or mental retardation. All pregnant women should therefore be advised not to eat undercooked meat and to find someone else to clean the cat litter tray.

TRAVEL VACCINES

The advice varies depending on the country you are visiting and even on whether you are visiting an urban or rural area. Don't depend on your travel agent to advise you. Most travel agents will try to give good advice but they are not provided with current recommendations as frequently as practice nurses who can give you the latest available advice. Children hate injections! Many parents book holidays without realising that vaccines are recommended so check with your nurse first.

➤ IMMUNISATIONS

UNDESCENDED TESTES

The testes or testicles develop inside the body and descend into the scrotum before birth. Baby boys are checked at birth and at eight weeks for undescended testes. If testes do not descend into the scrotum by themselves an operation may be needed to prevent problems in later life.

URINE INFECTION

➤ KIDNEY INFECTIONS

URTICARIA

Urticaria is an allergic condition which presents with a blotchy rash. The rash can resemble nettle stings. It is often due to food or drinks and may even be due to an additive, say, in a fizzy drink. We often have to wrack our brains to come up with the culprit but the treatment is usually straightforward – antihistamines (and avoidance of the culprit of course!).

VERRUCA

A verruca is a wart which develops on the sole of the foot and therefore it is usually flat. Most verrucae are not uncomfortable and so it is not fair to subject a child to painful treatment for a condition which will eventually get better by itself. If the verruca is causing pain then it can be treated either by applying salicylic acid every day (available from the pharmacist) or by freezing with liquid nitrogen or a similar substance at the surgery.

Most verrucae disappear after a year or two, are only very slightly infectious, and do not cause any harmful effects elsewhere on the body.

VIRUSES

Viruses are microscopic organisms which cause infection. There are millions of different types and many different strains of each type. Patients hoping for a quick prescription must get irritated by doctors telling them, 'It's just a virus' but it's usually true: viruses can cause fever, headache and muscle aches, sore throat, earache, hoarseness, coughs, swollen glands, rashes, tiredness, poor appetite, vomiting, diarrhoea, cold sores, joint pains, chest pains and many other symptoms!

There are few effective treatments for viral illnesses. Antibiotics do nothing unless a patient has developed a bacterial illness on top of their viral illness (for example, sinusitis after a cold). The drugs which are effective against viruses are used mainly in hospital and in patients who have poor resistance to infection because of other illnesses. Doctors are very cautious because they do not want to risk viruses becoming resistant to anti-viral drugs in the same way that bacteria have become resistant to antibiotics.

The good news is that otherwise healthy adults and children have a good natural defence against these organisms and the vast majority of viral illnesses will heal without causing damage to the tissues of the body.

What you can do...

• With viruses you treat the symptoms. Treat fever as described in the section on fever and treat pain with paracetamol.

• Call the doctor if there are any of the worrying signs listed in the section on fever.

• Doctors will not usually prescribe antibiotics unless there is a secondary bacterial infection.

VOMITING

Vomiting can be caused by many different illnesses in children. Almost any illness which causes a fever can cause vomiting. However the most common cause of prolonged vomiting which doctors see is gastro-enteritis.

In all cases of vomiting the main priority is maintaining a good intake of fluids. Even when vomiting is very persistent it is essential to keep encouraging a child to drink. Any fluid will do except for those which have large amounts of glucose, i.e. the high energy drinks and drinks which are very acidic such as fruit juices.

The next priority is the fever and this should be treated as advised above.

Signs of dehydration include a dry mouth or tongue, skin which has lost its elasticity, a sunken soft spot on the top of the head in a child under the age of 18 months and dry nappies. If you think your child has dehydration you should call your doctor. However it is unlikely that a child who has vomited once or twice has dehydration and doctors are unable to prescribe drugs to stop vomiting in young children.

➤ GASTRO-ENTERITIS

WARTS

➤ VERRUCA

WHOOPING COUGH

➤ CHILDHOOD FEVERS (PERTUSSIS)

WORMS

➤ THREADWORM

RESOURCES

Remember that your health visitor, who works from your GP's surgery, is your best professional friend. She will be able to help you with every kind of parenting problem, not just the medical ones. Even if she hasn't got the answer herself, she'll be able to put you in touch with someone who has – so try her first.

BREASTFEEDING
National Childbirth Trust
Alexandra House, Oldham Terrace
London W3 6NH
Tel: 0181 992 8637
Mon–Fri 9.30am–4.30pm
Ring them to ask for the phone number of your local breastfeeding counsellor. You don't have to join the NCT to get help.

Breastfeeding Network
Tel: 0870 900 8787
Independent support locally.

La Leche League (Great Britain)
BM 3424
London WC1N 3XX
Tel: 0171 242 1278
Breastfeeding help.

Association of Breastfeeding
Mothers (ABM)
Tel: 0171 813 1481
9am–5pm
Telephone support.

CRYING
Serene and the Cry-sis Helpline
Tel: 0171 404 5011
8am–11pm every day
Self-help and support for the parents and carers of excessively crying, sleepless, and demanding babies and young children.

A central answering service gives the names and phone numbers of fully-trained volunteers in your area to contact for support.

TWINS
Twins and Multiple Births
Association (TAMBA)
Harnott House
309 Chester Road
Little Sutton
Ellesmere Port CH66 1QQ
Tel: 0151 348 0020
Helpline: 01732 868000
Mon–Fri 7pm–11pm, and
10am–11pm at weekends.
Information and support for parents who are expecting (or who have) twins, triplets, or more.

Multiple Births Foundation
Tel: 0181 383 3519
Telephone counselling.

NAPPIES
National Association of Nappy
Services
Nappy Tales
Unit 1
Hall Farm
South Moreton
Oxon OX11 9AH
Tel: 0121 693 4949
Can put you in touch with a nappy service in your area.

WORK AND CHILDCARE
Parents At Work
45 Beech Street
London EC2Y 8AD
Tel: 0171 628 3578
Fax: 0171 628 3591
For advice and information on all childcare and employment issues relating to pregnancy and working parents.
An answering machine takes your call 24 hours a day. It gives out another number for personal attention, or you can leave your address for an information pack.

The Maternity Alliance
45 Beech Street
London EC2Y 8AD
Tel: 0171 588 8582
Fax: 0171 588 8584
Works for better health service provision before conception and during pregnancy, childbirth and the first year of life.

Daycare Trust
Shoreditch Town Hall Annexe
380 Old Street
London EC12 9LT
Tel: 0171 739 2866
Fax: 0171 739 5579
National childcare charity campaigning to improve conditions for the working parent.

National Childminding
Association (NCMA)
8 Masons Hill
Bromley
Kent BR2 9EY
Tel: 0181 464 6164
Helpline: 0181 466 0200
Mon–Tue 2–4pm,
Thurs 1–3pm
Fax: 0181 290 6834

PREMATURE BABIES
BLISS–Baby Life Support Systems
Tel: 0171 831 9393
BLISS provides support and a
listening ear to the parents and
families of 'special care' babies –
both in hospital and at home.

WHAT TO EAT?
Sainsbury's/Wellbeing
Eating for Pregnancy
Helpline 0114 242 4084
Mon–Fri 9am–4pm
Can also give advice on eating
while breastfeeding.

Vegan Society
7 Battle Road
St Leonards-on-Sea
East Sussex TN37 7AA
Tel: 01424 427393
Dietary advice and leaflets
available for vegan parents.

Vegetarian Society
Parkdale
Dunham Road
Altrincham
Cheshire WA14 4QG
Tel: 0161 928 0793
Support for vegetarian parents.

PARENTING
Gingerbread
16–17 Clerkenwell Close
London EC1R 0AA
Tel: 0171 336 8183
Help for one-parent families.

National Council for One-Parent
Families
255 Kentish Town Road
London NW5 2LX
Tel: 0171 267 1361
For financial and legal information
and referrals.

Parent Network
Tel: 0171 735 1214
Mon–Fri 10am–4pm
Runs local 'Parent-link' support
groups teaching parenting skills.

Parentline
Tel: 01702 559900
Helpline for parents under stress.

NEED FRIENDS?
The National Childbirth Trust
Tel: 0181 992 8637
Mon–Fri 9.30am–4.30pm
Can put you in touch with local
postnatal support groups.

Meet-A-Mum Association
Helpline 0181 768 0123
Mon–Fri 7pm–10pm
MAMA is a nationwide group that
puts mums into contact with
other mums in their region. They
also hold study days.

Association for Post-Natal Illness
(APNI)
25 Jerdan Place
London SW6 1BE
Tel: 0171 386 0868
Fax: 0171 386 8885
For mothers who are feeling very
depressed and need support.

Home-Start
2 Salisbury Road
Leicester LE1 7QR
Tel: 0116 233 9955
Trained volunteers will come to
your home and lend a hand when
you're under stress.

SPECIFIC PROBLEMS
Action for Sick Children
300 Kingston Road
Wimbledon Chase
London SW20 8LX
Tel: 0181 542 4848
Fax: 0181 542 2424
Advice and information for
parents with children in hospital.

Association for Spina Bifida and
Hydrocephalus
ASBAH House
42 Park Road
Peterborough PE1 2UQ
Tel: 01733 555988

British Diabetic Association
10 Queen Anne Street
London W1M 0BD
Careline 0171 636 6112
Mon–Fri 9am–5pm
Aims to help and care for people
with diabetes or those who are
close to them.

Cleft Lip and Palate Association
(CLAPA)
235–237 Finchley Road
London NW3 6LS
Tel: 0171 431 0033
Fax: 0171 431 8881

The Coeliac Society
PO Box 220
High Wycombe
Buckinghamshire HP11 2HY
Tel: 01494 437278

Contact-a-Family
Tel: 0171 383 3555
Helping families of children with
'special needs'.

Down's Syndrome Association
155 Mitcham Road
London SW17 9PG
Tel: 0181 682 4001
For children and carers.

Health Information Service
Tel: 0800 665544 (England and Wales)
Tel: 0800 224488 (Scotland)
Tel: 0345 581929 (N. Ireland)
Mon–Fri 10am–5pm
A national network of NHS-funded helplines providing free, confidential information on illnesses and treatments, rights and complaints. Around 200 lines covering 26 centres.

MIND
MINDINFOLINE 0345 660163
Mon–Fri 9.15am–4.45pm
A confidential mental health information service. Provides information, support, and understanding to callers.

Multiple Sclerosis Society
Helpline 0171 371 8000
Mon–Fri 10am–4pm, as well as Tues–Thurs 6–8pm
Five salaried staff and 15 trained volunteers answer calls on all aspects of multiple sclerosis.

ParentAbility
PO Box 72
Ruislip
Middlesex HA4 6XU
Peer network supporting disabled people becoming parents.

REACH
12 Wilson Way
Earl's Barton
Northamptonshire
NN6 0NZ
Tel: 01604 811041
The association for children with hand/arm deficiency.

SCOPE
6 Market Road
London N7 9PW
Tel: 0171 619 7100

Helpline: 0800 626216
Mon–Fri 11am–9pm
Sat–Sun 2–6pm
Fax: 0171 436 2601
Help for children with cerebral palsy and their carers.

Sickle Cell Society
54 Station Road
Harlesden
London NW10 4UA
Tel: 0181 961 7795
or 0181 961 4006
Fax: 0181 961 8346

SMOKING
Quitline 0800 002200
Every day 9am–11pm
Telephone counselling for those who are trying to stop smoking, in a wide variety of languages. Can also put you in touch with local support groups.

COT DEATH
Foundation for the Study of Infant Deaths (FSID)
14 Halkin Street
London SW1X 7DP
Tel: 0171 235 0965
Helpline: 0171 235 1721 (24 hour)
Works to prevent sudden infant death and promote infant health by funding research, supporting bereaved families, and providing information to the general public.

BACK
General Osteopathic Council
Tel: 0171 357 6655
A recorded message will give you an option to select for the Osteopathic Information Service – for further information about osteopathy and details of osteopaths in your area. They can also help you find a registered practitioner of cranial osteopathy.

FURTHER READING
NCT Publishing has produced the following useful and informative pregnancy and childcare titles:

Being Pregnant, Giving Birth
Mary Nolan
You and Your New Baby
Anna McGrail
Breastfeeding Your Baby
Jane Moody, Jane Britten, and Karen Hogg
Working Parents' Companion
Teresa Wilson

also
NCT Book of Antenatal Tests
Mary Nolan
NCT Book of Postnatal Depression
Heather Welford
NCT Book of First Foods
Ravinder Lilly
NCT Book of Potty Training
Heather Welford
NCT Book of Crying Baby
Anna McGrail
NCT Book of Sleep
Penney Hames
NCT Book of Safe Foods
Hannah Hulme Hunter and Rosemary Dodds

– all published by Thorsons in collaboration with National Childbirth Trust Publishing Ltd.

INDEX